Interstitial Cystitis:
A Personal Journey of COMPLETE Healing!

Tracy Alexis, PhD

BALBOA.
PRESS

A DIVISION OF HAY HOUSE

Balboa Press books may be ordered through booksellers or by contacting:

Balboa Press
A Division of Hay House
1663 Liberty Drive
Bloomington, IN 47403
www.balboapress.com
1 (877) 407-4847

Because of the dynamic nature of the Internet, any web addresses or links contained in this book may have changed since publication and may no longer be valid. The views expressed in this work are solely those of the author and do not necessarily reflect the views of the publisher, and the publisher hereby disclaims any responsibility for them.

The author of this book does not dispense medical advice or prescribe the use of any technique as a form of treatment for physical, emotional, or medical problems without the advice of a physician, either directly or indirectly. The intent of the author is only to offer information of a general nature to help you in your quest for emotional and spiritual well-being. In the event you use any of the information in this book for yourself, which is your constitutional right, the author and the publisher assume no responsibility for your actions.

Scripture quotations are taken from the Holy Bible, New International Version®, NIV®. Copyright © 1973, 1978, 1984, 2011 by Biblica, Inc.™ Used by permission of Zondervan. All rights reserved worldwide. www.zondervan.com The "NIV" and "New International Version" are trademarks registered in the United States Patent and Trademark Office by Biblica, Inc.™

Print information available on the last page.

ISBN: 978-1-9822-3222-1 (sc)
ISBN: 978-1-9822-3224-5 (hc)
ISBN: 978-1-9822-3223-8 (e)

Library of Congress Control Number: 2019910738

Balboa Press rev. date: 10/03/2019

Testimonials

"Tracy Alexis is a medical super hero! In this powerful book filled with essential information, Dr. Alexis not only presents her personal experience of how she achieved remission from Interstitial Cystitis within five years, but also explains how she navigated the Scylla and Charybdis of commercial insurance bureaucracy, medical negligence, and "support group" stagnation. Readers will certainly learn about Interstitial Cystitis, and its effective and ineffective interventions, but perhaps more importantly, they will learn how one patient's indomitable spirit and curiosity propelled a successful journey of healing. I predict this story will motivate, inspire, and hopefully, transform the lives of patients and medical professionals alike."

—Grace E. Jackson, M.D.
Sedona, AZ

"Dr. Alexis has produced a thoroughly comprehensive and intimate portrait of Interstitial Cystitis (IC) for which I am grateful. Her clarity of vision has fanned away the fog that has kept this condition in obscurity and brought it into the daylight. A decade and a half as a pharmacist have not given me the kind of detailed knowledge that this book provides. My hope is that its distribution will facilitate understanding and empathy in the medical community for the underserved population and provide guidance for those who suffer needlessly."

—David Wales, PharmD, RPh
Albuquerque, NM

"Thoroughly researched and well written, this book provides the reader with guidance, direction, and helpful specifics presented compassionately and didactically through self-disclosure and factual information. Dr. Alexis addresses all aspects of her healing journey and provides sound advice while remaining cognizant of individual differences. A must-read for anyone suffering from or associated in any way with Interstitial Cystitis or related issues. I have indeed found it a meaningful resource for general medical purposes as well."

—David Brendel, PhD
Los Angeles, CA

Note To Readers

This book contains the opinions and ideas of its author. It is intended to provide helpful and informative material on the subjects it addresses. It is sold with the understanding that the author and publisher are not engaged in rendering medical, health, psychiatric, psychological, or any other kind of personal professional services in the book. Readers should consult their medical, health, psychiatric, psychological, or other competent professional before adopting any of the suggestions in this book or drawing inferences from it.

The author and publisher specifically disclaim all responsibility for any liability, loss, or risk, personal or otherwise, which is incurred as a consequence, directly or indirectly, of the use and application of any of the contents of this book.

Dedication

This book is dedicated to every individual who suffers from Interstitial Cystitis, fibromyalgia, chronic inflammation, or other mysterious illnesses for which traditional medicine states "there are no known etiologies" and, thus, no known cures. This book is also for those who lack trust in today's medical systems, licensed providers, mammoth, and prosperous insurance companies.

For those who suffer from trauma-related maladies or ailments, may you each find meaningful healing help within the pages of this book.

Contents

Foreword

When Tracy Alexis and I met 11 years ago, she had already developed a distinguished reputation in our state for her competence and enthusiasm in her work with the underprivileged. At that time I was dedicating a considerable amount of my practice to the examination of applicants for social security disability benefits, and that is how our paths crossed. Soon after that meeting, we were both receiving prestigious awards for our respective professional efforts—I for my work with the so-called mentally ill as well as for serving as the co-editor-in-chief of a psychological journal—and she in recognition of her passion for helping those less fortunate. Tracy saw this coincidence as encouragement to pursue a PhD in Industrial/Organizational Psychology with me as her academic advisor. I agreed, and the rest, as they say, is history. This book is part of that history.

A few years into our academic relationship, Tracy was involved in a serious motorcycle accident. A year or so later, she experienced a complete bladder death as well as the manifestation of other trauma-related symptoms, eventually leading her to a diagnosis of Interstitial Cystitis (IC). Few local physicians or specialists had even heard of this disease, and even fewer had ever seen a case so severe or had successfully treated IC cases.

Tracy's attempts to find competent help are a part of this story, but the most important part of her book is the extent to which she discovered—through her own research and self-experimentation (using the single-case experimental designs she had employed during her doctoral dissertation)—how the painful and debilitating symptoms of Interstitial Cystitis and other inflammatory diseases including fibromyalgia could be effectively treated and healed. (Single-case experimental designs are real science, leading to the ability to predict and even control illnesses, as opposed to statistical analyses of groups of patients whose conclusions change before the ink is dry on journalists' uncritical reports of them.)

This book is an intensely personal but balanced account of Dr. Alexis' journey through the maze of traditional, expensive, and largely ineffective medical interventions to much more gentle, humane, and effective approaches and solutions. I feel confident that the techniques she offers in this book will undoubtedly be accepted into alternative medicine.

There are those among us scientists who might assert that some of what she says in this book goes against "established medical facts." Perhaps so, but my view is that the history of medicine, as well as the history of other scientific fields, is strewn with the remains of so-called established facts. Indeed, the American philosopher Hilary Putnam has suggested that the previously asserted solid distinction between fact and value is collapsing.

Tracy has taught me through her experiences with the medical establishment that people—professionals as well as lay people—will believe what it suits their purposes to believe, *regardless of the data,* and that too much of their purpose is to make money and achieve prestige and position at the expense of the hapless public. I hope that one day traditionally trained physicians will incorporate alternative medicine—which is much like the traditional Eastern medical approach—into their practice and see Dr. Alexis' work in particular as no threat to the views traditional American physicians espouse.

Health statistics suggest that as much as 10% of the entire world's population suffers from Interstitial Cystitis. That's a lot of people who could benefit from the recommendations in this small but powerful book!

Louis Wynne, PhD
Clinical Psychologist

Acknowledgements

It is with great humility and a depth of gratitude that is challenging to convey that I wish to acknowledge the individuals who have assisted with the edits and finalization of this book.

Louis Wynne, PhD, my graduate studies academic advisor, for his motivational speeches, truthfulness, clinical and scientific expertise, behavioral insights, unwavering professional expectations, and undying friendship, even in light of my frequent and overt resistance to his suggested language inclusions, exclusions and/or modifications—I cannot thank you enough … and this book publication satisfies my post-doctorial debt.

To ALL who helped by proofreading and suggesting revisions to make the flow and ease of understanding this book better for my readers, however significant or modest those suggestions might have been, I thank you humbly and sincerely for your time, candor, and shared perceptions to help me get from concept to this finalized version of a printed copy!

Dr. Bruce (you know who you are), thank you for your medical insights and expertise, without which the more relevant and esoteric scientific truths of my medical journey might not have been understandable. Doubtless, without your extremely thoughtful input, the medical and self-help aspects of this book would never have been transformed into a sensible layperson format, which was always my overarching goal.

Sandra McGinnis, you were so wonderful to tease apart the supplements section of my initial manuscript, which you can see now, was appropriately reunited with the story of my healing journey. Thank you for your constructively critical feedback about where to expand my writing, what to eliminate altogether, and for your limitless patience in helping me understand more as a writer about all of the necessary components a reader might seek from this book, as well as for your thoughtful and continuous edits. My appreciation to you is heartfelt and enduring.

For all who took time from their very busy lives to read my draft manuscript and offer their input, suggestions, comments—both negative and positive—and for your reinforcing feedback, I am deeply grateful. Tim Shroyer, Pamela Chavez, David Wales, as well as those mentioned above and below this paragraph ...thank you, each!

To my very dear friend, John Cline of John Cline Productions, for his consistent patience, cogent technical knowledge, amazing photography skills, and salient business acumen, my appreciation is lifelong and limitless.

Lastly, to the pastors of my church—Copper Pointe Church in Albuquerque, New Mexico—the Galen Woodward

Family, thank you for motivating me to fulfill my dream of finishing this project. There were numerous times I was so overwhelmed that I could not focus or make meaningful headway, but your uncanny on-point sermons full of divine encouragement helped me re-center, re-focus, and realize that this book *is* an important piece of my God-given destiny. With an openly grateful heart, I thank each of you!

Dreams are so much easier to manifest into reality with such supportive friends, colleagues, and advisors. My genuine and heartfelt gratitude to each and every one listed above, as well as the many IC sufferers with whom I interacted during my healing journey for helping me achieve this dream. Thank you. Thank you. Thank you!

"You can be broken into a dozen shattered pieces and still heal the world because service has its own medicine – hope." – Shannon L. Alder

Introduction

Like most Americans, I had never heard of Interstitial Cystitis (IC). No one among my relatives, my colleagues, or other acquaintances had ever been afflicted by IC. But then, in late 2009, I began to have excruciating pains in my abdomen. The first physician who examined me diagnosed my condition as a urinary tract infection (UTI). However, I had experienced UTIs before, and the pain I was experiencing was vastly different from the pain of a UTI! A second physician and then a third were equally confounded. Physicians, as many Americans soon find out to their dismay, are not as smart, especially as diagnosticians, as all those TV commercials try to convince us they are.

I had been thrown off my motorcycle and slammed onto the street a few months earlier by a pickup truck that crashed into me. The pickup had been hit on the other side by an automobile that failed to stop for a red traffic light, pushing the truck into my lane and causing impact with my motorcycle, creating the crash that up-ended my life. When my symptoms developed, and as they grew worse over time, I became confident that my debilitating IC was caused by the motorcycle wreck, despite that doctors do not know or understand the causes (etiology) of IC.

In order to be accepted as a *disease*, four criteria (developed by Rudolf Ludwig Carl Virchow in 1847[1]) must be met. Those four criteria are: symptoms; pathology; course; and etiology.

The first criterion is that the disease must have consistent symptoms. People who have the supposed illness must display similar symptoms. In the case of IC, this would be painful urination, frequent urination, and a dysfunctional bladder but there might be other symptoms as well. Physicians know the *symptomology* of IC and they think they know the *tissue pathology* but they do not yet know the *course* or the *etiology*. Within the medical community there is considerable disagreement, especially regarding the etiology of IC. The question of etiology is crucial, and it concerns many, if not most, other diseases as well.

It may come as a surprise to the readers of this book that medical professionals do not know the etiology (cause) of many of the diseases from which we suffer: essential hypertension, fibromyalgia (which I also developed immediately after my motorcycle wreck and which has vanished miraculously with the approaches outlined in this book), endometriosis, Hashimoto's disease, lupus, Graves' disease, Crohn's disease and irritable bowel syndrome, GERD, types 1 and 2 diabetes, etc. Indeed, many of the recommendations made in this book are widely applicable to other diseases, as well, *especially* fibromyalgia, of which I cured myself.

Most of the time, physicians just say that they don't know what ails us, and then they fall back on family history as a means to try to discover the possible causes of our discomfort. For example, if every woman in your family has suffered from breast cancer, you probably will too. *But that is conjecture, **not** etiology!* A conclusion reached in that manner is mere coincidence or crude extrapolation. One must still answer the questions: *Why* did every woman in the family have this disease and, if any did not, why didn't she?

Some of medicine's answers to the etiology question are quaint but they are never amusing because they have led to practices that border on the barbaric. Consider, for examples, blood-letting in the not-too-distant past as a treatment that was reputed to have shortened George Washington's life, or lobotomies as a treatment for schizophrenia.

My diagnosis of IC was not reached immediately; in fact, I first had to endure various medical professionals' conjectures and speculations, in addition to listening to the many physicians tell me (and treat me as if), "You've just got a *common* urinary tract infection." Too many of those physicians, para-professionals, nurses, and other health care specialists, when they had heard of IC, had no direct experience with it. Even less could any of them recommend a successful treatment. Indeed, it may be through learning what treatments work that medical science will learn the etiology of IC.

It must also be said that many physicians are not even remotely interested in the etiology of the diseases they treat.

Their view is that knowing whatever works in alleviating pain is all they need to know. This pain relief is in fact called *palliative care* (care that eliminates/reduces a patient's pain) but I call its underlying theory *miasmic*.

Barely a hundred years ago it was generally believed by the medical profession that diseases such as measles, whooping cough, scarlet fever, and diphtheria were caused by miasmas: invisible and odorless gases that seeped up through the ground at night and infected unsuspecting pedestrians. Many of the great-grandparents of this book's readers felt that "the night air was dangerous," as if to say that the air at night was somehow different from the air during the day. What was sold to the public as medical fact in those days is regarded as superstitious nonsense today.

Discovering an illness' etiology is extremely difficult work and often involves the study of generations (that's why doctors ask for family histories), and the results are rarely welcomed. For example, there is strong evidence that many diseases which have made their appearances known since around 1960 might be the result of the patient's mother having been exposed to persistent endocrine-disrupting chemicals if she lived near a Superfund site during her pregnancy. To demonstrate this theory conclusively, as is the case in so many medical instances, would upset the legal departments of a lot of industrial corporations. (For example, watch the film *Erin Brockovich*[2].)

It became very clear that I was on my own, then, when it came to *successfully* healing my IC. This book tells the story of the treatments I received, my own discoveries to help heal my body, as well as which treatments and self-discoveries worked and which did not—including which treatments at the hands of medical professionals made my bladder situation even worse.

My symptoms will be described as they developed, waxed, and waned. I will recount my efforts to seek help, discuss the help that I did receive, and, finally, share what—thanks largely to my own efforts—did the most to relieve my symptoms.[3]

I hasten to add that I do not mean to disparage all physicians. Far from it! The physicians and staff at University of New Mexico Hospital, specifically those in the uro-gynecology (uro-gyn) clinic (the clinic devoted exclusively to urologic issues that plague females) were extremely helpful and detailed in their treatment approach, and I thank them now, especially Dr. Yoku Komesu, for all they did to help me heal my dysfunctional bladder. But others at different hospitals and medical facilities, where I was required to submit myself for treatments because my health care insurance changed over the years, were not helpful! More on that later. I hope that you, as a sufferer of IC (and fibromyalgia or other chronic inflammatory diseases), are as lucky in your search for help as I eventually was!

This book does make representations of some concepts such as chemistry, biochemistry, physiology, metabolism, and nutraceutical (a food containing health-giving additives and having medicinal benefit) as *established* facts, and these representations deviate from what science and/or scientists may regard as valid.

"Beware of false knowledge; it is more dangerous than ignorance." – George Bernard Shaw

Chapter 1

Background, Context, and Medical History

As much as 10% of the world's population suffers from Interstitial Cystitis[4] (IC), a chronic inflammatory[*] bladder condition that causes frequent and often painful urination. IC is sometimes called painful bladder syndrome (PBS) or bladder pain syndrome (BPS).

The bladder is a balloon in which urine is retained after it leaves the kidneys through the ureters. Once a significant amount of urine is deposited in the bladder, the urinary sphincter muscle triggers the release of urine so it can exit the body. The bladder is the active participant in this process. At the beginning of my IC, I felt like my urine was on fire. Any urine I was able to pass created a pinching

---

[*] Many conditions that were once taught to physicians as "autoimmune" have been re-conceptualized as mainly inflammatory (e.g., allergy, asthma, coeliac (a/k/a celiac) disease, glomerulonephritis, hepatitis, inflammatory bowel disease, transplant rejection). Medicine cannot yet alter a patient's immune system, however; it can attempt to reduce a patient's inflammation.

sensation in my urethra (the tube through which the urine exits and goes outside the body), and the drips and dribbles of passing urine felt like burning gasoline. Physiologically, I experienced a constant sharp, stabbing pain in my lower left pelvis that remained for several years—even a soft, gentle touch in that lower left pelvic area made me howl in agony. I later learned that the pain in the lower left pelvis area was referred pain caused by nerves that were near the actual trauma area, "referring" discomfort elsewhere in my body.

I learned that many people who have IC experience painful, debilitating symptoms endlessly while others may have periods of pain dotted by random stretches of time without any discomfort whatsoever. Physicians do not know why this variation occurs, but conjecture that it may have to do with the severity of bladder damage in each patient. Medical providers do not even know how to diagnose IC because there is no scientifically agreed-upon etiology.

Unfortunately for sufferers, when medical professionals are uncertain of the cause of an ailment or disease, they are equally as uncertain of how to treat that ailment or disease. However, one of the most common symptoms of IC is urinary pain that lasts for more than six weeks and is not caused by another bladder condition such as kidney stones or urinary tract infections.

Urinary pain that persists for any length of time brings about a special set of challenges that revolve around the need to empty one's bladder anywhere from 50 to 75, or more, times per day. Obviously, such frequent urination with its sensations of burning, stinging, and even pinching makes a decent night's sleep, travel, and productive employment nearly impossible.

Common sensations suffered by patients with IC are bladder pressure that becomes more and more uncomfortable as the bladder fills up, discomfort or pain in the urethra (the tube that transports urine from the bladder to the outside of the body), and the feeling that one needs to void again immediately after one has just gone.

This feeling to void again immediately after one has just gone should not be confused with what specialists call "double-voiding." Double-voiding is voiding a noticeable quantity of urine immediately after having *just* voided a significant quantity of urine. Typically, the IC sufferer voids as much as s/he is holding in her/his bladder but sometimes not all of the urine is emptied from the bladder and one must void again immediately after the first void, thus the term "double-voiding."

There may be another IC commonality, that of bladder ulcers. Bladder ulcers can bleed and, if they do, blood will appear in the urine. Blood in the urine creates an environment where bacteria grows and flourishes. Blood in the bladder is the underlying cause of a urinary tract infection (UTI)—a source of real misery!

Most of my physicians, nurse practitioners, and health care providers appeared genuinely concerned with my discomfort and seemed that they truly wanted to eliminate my pain.

Nevertheless, I couldn't get out of my mind the remark that one of my physician-friends shared with me: "The first thing we physicians learn in medical school is: Don't let a patient leave your office unless they feel you have done something to help them." I can't tell you how many times I left a physician's or specialist's office feeling that s/he had no idea what I was going through nor how to ensure I felt *helped* before my exit from their office. Countless times would be an understatement.

At one specialist's office I visited to try to discover what was wrong with my bladder, there was a large sign saying, "One detailed health history is worth a hundred tests." Unfortunately, the urologist there didn't follow his own posted admonition; he seemed extremely uninterested in my bladder health history and poo-pooed the history I shared, at least part of which I believed caused the discomfort that brought me to his office in the first place.

It did not help anyone connect the dots to my IC dilemma that more than a year elapsed between the *cause*—the physical trauma[5] I experienced from my motorcycle accident—and the *effect*—the development of my IC symptoms. This does not mean that serious medical issues were not developing within my body during that year, only that whatever tissue pathology was starting had not yet produced the full onset of misery that caused my bladder's death. Perhaps another woman of the same age might have felt pain months earlier, or months later. These differences from one patient to another are the enigmas of IC.

This attests to the fact of *"why"* research on human health problems—both medical and psychological—is so difficult. Research can take generations before important information is fleshed out, as the late Theo Colburn noted in her book *Our Stolen Future.*[6] Dr. Colburn noted that to connect the dots between (a) exposure of fetuses in-utero to industrial pollutants such as persistent endocrine-disrupting chemicals and (b) cancers in our reproductive organs, does not occur over a short period of time. Consider also that the spate of mass shootings in the 2000s and 2010s might well be the result of young men being raised in homes of absent fathers—a phenomenon that came into existence in the late 1960s and early 70s as divorce rates soared in the U.S. and single-mother-child-rearing households became quite commonplace.[7]

In the same way, the details of my motorcycle accident did not seem to matter medically until I realized that my body was not working the way it had been, and that I was not yet at the age in life to have the kind of body failure I was experiencing.

Without warning, then, during Thanksgiving weekend in 2010, my bladder totally and completely stopped working—it died! It shut down and would not do what it was designed to do, that is, release urine from my body. I had a house-full of guests visiting me for the holiday and, early in the evening, I felt the urge to empty my bladder. However, in the bathroom upon attempting to go, nothing came out. Nothing. Not even a drop.

Imagine my surprise, my concern, and the crushing fear I experienced when I could not void. There was no warning whatsoever … no urinary tract infection that led up to my bladder's death. Quite literally, one minute my bladder was totally okay and working just fine, and the next minute it wasn't!

The only thought I had was that it was a holiday weekend; physicians were scarce, and specialists even scarcer. I knew that even if I went to a hospital emergency room, my chances of getting any immediate relief were remote at best. Previous attempts to access emergency help when I had UTIs and pain emptying my bladder had resulted in a round of antibiotics and bladder anti-inflammatory pills that turned my urine a neon orange color.

Remembering what had been of some help in the past, I turned on the sink faucet to see whether hearing the water trickle would help start my stream of urine. It did not.

The only other action I thought might help was to get in the shower and feel warm water on my skin, hoping that would get my stream going. Fortunately, the guests I was entertaining understood and they were extremely gracious about my unexpected need to shower that evening. Thankfully they excused my uncharacteristically odd behavior.

Luckily, standing in the warm shower did get my stream of urine flowing again, but urine only trickled out. Clearly, my bladder wasn't working the way it had prior to this *death*.

Aside from an occasional bout with a UTI, I never had problems emptying my bladder. Once, 40 years ago when I was pregnant with my daughter, I had difficulty emptying my bladder, which led to a pretty severe UTI. My mother took me to her urologist because I had not previously experienced a UTI. Since I was pregnant, prescription medications were certainly not a treatment option. The urologist took a look inside my body and apparently, my urethra contained what he called "strictures"—little flaps of skin lining my urethra that prevented my urine from completely emptying from my bladder. Because of these strictures, a small amount of urine would remain in my bladder after I urinated, and those remaining few drops created bacterial growth in my bladder, which blossomed into a full-blown UTI.

The indicated remedy was to remove the strictures but, again, because I was pregnant, my options for post-removal pain medications were limited to Tylenol. The urologist administered a local anesthetic topically like novocaine, marcaine or lidocaine to numb me so that he could burn off (cauterize) the strictures. After this mostly non-eventful procedure, the urologist cautioned me that these strictures could grow back over a period of time and strongly suggested that I monitor the frequency of future UTIs, which might serve as an indicator that the strictures had re-grown. The cauterizing procedure was basically a minor outpatient surgery. I will return to discuss these strictures later in the book.

In my quest to get my bladder working again after the Thanksgiving holiday weekend, I attempted a "walk-in" visit at a urologist's clinic the first thing the following Monday morning without a referral from my primary care physician (PCP). However, the urologist would not see me without a referral from my PCP. At that point, I called my PCP, made an appointment with him for the earliest available opening, and received an appointment to see him fairly quickly. It was, however, with great difficulty that I produced the required urine sample for the PCP referral visit, which revealed some blood in my urine as well as an extremely high white blood cell count (characteristic of UTIs). Upon his discovery of my urine sample results, my PCP provided me with the requisite referral for a urologist's consultation.

"Doctors are men who prescribe medicine of which they know little, to cure diseases of which they know less, in human beings of which they know nothing." – Voltaire

Chapter 2

The Ugly Truth About Health Care And Its Providers

Several days came and went from the day I received the primary care provider referral until the day I was able to attend the scheduled urologist's appointment. During this delay, my bladder was not improving. However, before continuing with what took place when I did see the urologist, I want to draw your attention to the consequences for treatment of any organ that is situated deep within our bodies—and all of our organs are situated deep within our bodies. The bladder cannot be treated topically or with medication applied directly to the malfunctioning organ, as with other parts of the body like the skin, cornea of the eye, the middle ear, or the rectum which can be treated topically or by directly applying medication.

The bladder is treated by urologists who may put medication into the bladder through a catheter. This procedure of putting medication into the bladder through a catheter is called an "instillation." Once an instillation is received, the medication is held inside the bladder for 30 minutes, allowing the instilled medicines to bathe the bladder walls. Those medications are then passed out of the bladder in the usual way. More information on instillations is offered in Chapter 6.

The first urologist I saw for my IC was certainly not the last! I was seen by various physicians resulting in a mixed bag of ideas, treatments, as well as hoped-for and promised outcomes. Treatment by several different physicians was necessary as both my economic circumstances and my health insurance coverage shifted and changed over the course of time, yet it became very quickly apparent that the majority of physicians I went to were unable to help me. There was one exception: The local university hospital was the ONLY specialty clinic in my city that had an effective IC treatment program, treatment protocol *and* technique proficiency providing bladder instillations.

I use the term "treatment" in this book to mean so much more than the typical treatment a patient receives from the typical physician. Treatment here means both a treatment protocol, e.g., a prescription, but it also means treatment of the patient (in this instance *me*) with dignity and respect, *and* as an important *equal* co-participant in the journey to heal the body. I was extremely fortunate in that the specialists and physicians in the local hospital female-focused clinic engaged me and respected me as that *equal* co-participant in my IC healing. In exchange, I revered their expertise, their compassion, their obedience to the Hippocratic Oath, and the pleasantly unexpected *extras* of their human kindness and empathy.

It was immediately obvious that the treatment by the fee-for-service specialists was much more difficult to obtain due to the requirements of behemoth insurance-regulated health care systems. To access the insurance-regulated fee-for-service specialists, I needed a referral from my primary health care provider and I was required to see the specialists who were "in network." Just to establish myself as a patient in these fee-for-service systems, I was required to make an appointment, pay a co-pay fee, complete patient intake paperwork, ALL without *any* expectation whatsoever that a medical *service* (or comforting/palliative procedure) would be provided to me until such time as *they* determined I was an *established patient.*

A highly discomforting reality was when I was forced to receive instillations from a urologist (in name only) who had *never, ever* performed an instillation in his entire medical career. Upon learning that a treatment I had become intimately familiar with (from the numerous successful instillations I received at the University of New Mexico Hospital's Uro-Gyn Clinic) was "new" to him was anything *but* a confidence-builder! It was after these extremely painful experiences of literally being a *brand new* provider's *guinea pig* that I decided if my bladder was to be healed and its performance improved, I must take that healing into my own hands.

As time passed, I was bounced back-and-forth from free health care (which proved to me to be the best in my community) to the behemoth fee-for-service insured health care providers, which repeatedly and consistently demonstrated itself disappointingly inferior to the almost free stuff. Through these back-and-forth movements from one health care provider to another, I very quickly discovered that the so-called specialists for whom I had to pay through my fee-for-service insured health care coverage, were highly incompetent to help me (you will discover why when you read my complaint letter under the "self-advocacy" chapter in this book [Chapter 9]). Worse, when attempting to share information about the instillation technique to these incompetents, they wanted no input from me regarding what size catheter to use to perform the same identical procedure I had been receiving routinely (and practically free) from the professionals at the university hospital who knew what they were doing, and more importantly, *how to do it*! (The greater the number of the catheter, the larger its diameter. As a petite female, I needed a size 10 neonatal [baby] catheter … but more on this topic under "self-catherization" in Chapter 6.)

While we are on the topic of catheter size: The larger the catheter, the greater chance it may create additional scar tissue[8] in the urethra during insertion, which—in addition to creating unnecessary pain—exacerbates IC and prevents healing.

Additionally, the incompetent, unprofessional hospital staff (who had *never* performed an instillation) frequently disagreed vehemently with each other, in open view—behaviors I found to be not only highly unprofessional but also devoid of creating a sense of calm about having them put objects necessary for an instillation inside my body. When I told the urologist to whom my PCP had referred me about the 30-plus-year-ago cauterization of strictures from my urethra, he snorted and said, "No physician would perform such a barbaric procedure!" I thought it wise to *not* point out that the history of medicine has demonstrated a considerable degree of barbaric practices, such as blood-letting to rid the body of ailments (which dates back millennia) and psychiatry's electroconvulsive shock therapy and deep brain stimulation that are more recent evidences of medicine's barbaric practices, hence, Hippocrates' oath that physicians "First, do no harm!"

Given that this urologist and I weren't exactly establishing an amicable doctor-patient relationship, I literally had to beg him to humor me and conduct a cystoscope to reassure me that my previously removed strictures had not re-grown in my urethra. (A cystoscope is a tiny camera that is inserted into the bladder through a catheter and provides the urologist a view of what is happening inside the bladder.) Very reluctantly, he agreed, and his tiny camera showed us that the strictures had not re-grown, yet it did reveal something else medically unpleasant.

To quickly dismiss me from his office upon this unpleasant discovery, this urologist prescribed tamsulosin, whose trade name is Flomax—which I was to find out later is *not* FDA-approved as a treatment of IC. After taking Flomax for almost a year, it did restore my bladder's function, but I learned that

I had significantly diminished bladder capacity. Prior to my bladder's death, I had about a 16-ounce bladder capacity; after my bladder functions were restored, I barely had an ounce of bladder capacity. As the urologist was tearing off the completed prescription from the pad of empty ones, he rather matter-of-factly told me that the cystoscope revealed my bladder displayed large mast cells, which he went on to state, with no attempt at professional decorum or bedside manner whatsoever, "…is an indicator of **bladder cancer**"! Imagine my alarm at hearing the cancer word. What was worse was that he could not wait to dismiss me from his office very matter-of-factly so that he could check in on his next patient. Later, I learned through my research for this book, that mast cells are also indicators of—and present with—IC!

This concluded my first, but certainly not my last, interaction with a specialist who was totally clueless about what I had or how to treat it.

One of the first things the physicians at the local university hospital uro-gyn clinic did was take me off the tamsulosin before they began providing me with fabulous and frequent instillations that were so soothing and healing to my bladder.

It was here, at University of New Mexico Hospital's Uro-Gyn Clinic that I learned the go-to oral medication prescribed by physicians to treat the symptoms of IC is pentosan polysulfate sodium (commonly called Elmiron). Many IC sufferers—including me—find this drug sickeningly toxic, resulting in all manner of unwanted and unpleasant side effects. I ingested only one dose (and can't imagine anyone taking it three times each day as the treatment protocol requires) and I suffered nausea, diarrhea, vomiting, raging headaches, severe hair loss, unusual and prolonged bruising (which I still experience six years after taking that single dose), blurred vision, and tinnitus, as the major side effects—but other ill-effects as well, all from taking just one pill!

A brief note on medication side effects: You certainly know that all drugs have a lengthy list of effects, but which are main effects and which are side effects is *entirely arbitrary.* One could argue that the main effects of pentosan polysulfate sodium are nausea, diarrhea, unusual bruising, severe hair loss, etc., and the side-effect is (hopefully) some relief from the symptoms of IC. You can get an education in unwanted and dangerous drug side effects just by listening to the dozens of medication advertisements aired daily on public television. The last I heard, the United States and New Zealand are the only countries in the entire world that permit drug merchandising directly to the public through mass media.

Since this book also discusses diet as one of the main elements in my treatment program for healing IC, I will note here that one of the best-kept secrets in America today is that our epidemic of obesity is not caused by sugar, or by the lack of exercise, or even by our high carbohydrate intake— although these certainly play a part—*but by the widespread consumption of prescription medications that have a side effect of weight gain.*

I decided, as a result of my experiences with fee-for-service physician incompetence performing instillations, as well as their propensity for prescribing toxic medications, to take my healing into my own hands. My training as a behavioral scientist (I have a PhD in Industrial/Organizational psychology) taught me, first, to observe my symptoms without any preconceived ideas about what their etiology might be; second, to hold in abeyance any hypothesis medical professionals and I might conjecture regarding how my symptoms developed; and finally, to test what the "causative" factors were by using a single-case model with an A-B-A-B design in which A is the baseline; B is one of the contributing factors; A2 is the regeneration of the baseline; and B2 is now re-imposed as the "treatment." This approach actually worked well towards my own healing.

I began by scrutinizing every aspect of my life to learn what was making my IC worse and what I had within my own control to make my IC better. I examined my diet, my employment, my stress level (stress creates cortisol, which causes the body's pH to become more acidic from the increased glucose secretion), my intake of herbal supplements, my exercise regimen, and how much rest I was or was not getting, etc. All of these variables were consistently reviewed, re-reviewed and incorporated into my (generally) self-directed healing program.

"Heal me, Oh Lord, and I will be healed...."
– Jeremiah 17:14 [NIV]

Chapter 3

My Basic "Healing" Tool Kit!

Through research and scrutiny, I devised a *basic* treatment regimen that consisted of four dietary supplements I call *my basic "healing" tool kit*. Throughout this book I will mention dietary supplements available from a particular manufacturer or reference them by specific brand name. Providing you—the reader—the specific manufacturer or brand name of a product is not intended as an endorsement or a recommendation that you purchase any of these products from any specific retailer or manufacturer. I have no connection or "skin in the game": meaning, I receive no benefits (monetary, personal, employment, consultative, etc.) of any kind from any of these supplement purveyors.

I emphasize that you should *always consult with your physician prior* to incorporating new supplements into your diet or intake. A supplement's interaction, positive or adverse, with medications you have been prescribed and are regularly taking is always possible. Your primary care physician or other medical specialist, e.g., urologist, gynecologist, oncologist, is aware of your health, what medications you are taking, and what your body might be lacking in the form of nutrients and s/he should know if there are any contra-indications for you to consider before incorporating new supplements. In addition, you should seriously consider not only monitoring what you add (and subtract) to (and from) your diet but you should keep a journal of when and in what amounts you made any changes (additions or deletions of a supplement, food, beverage, exercise, etc.). Keeping a journal will assist you going forward.[9]

There were basically FOUR products that I used daily to ensure my IC and any IC flares, stayed far away from me. This is my fundamental or *my basic "healing" tool kit.*

Again, as a behaviorist, I approached my healing from very deliberate research and scrutinizing frames of reference. With that stated, please recall that early in my treatment before a real diagnosis had been given to me, I suffered recurring urinary tract infections (UTIs). Those "historical" UTIs cleared up with a round of antibiotics. But my UTI experiences I had with my IC diagnosis would return immediately as the round of antibiotics were completed. This (returning UTI later diagnosed as IC) went on for ten solid months! And, it was the recurring UTIs that ultimately "told" my specialty care diagnosticians what my bladder was experiencing was *more and worse* than a UTI. However, because I had taken at least 10 separate rounds of antibiotics in as many months, I knew my digestive tract had been completely destroyed. Antibiotics are designed to kill bacteria. Unfortunately, antibiotics cannot "select" which bacteria they kill. Antibiotics kill bad bacteria as well as the good bacteria which reside in our digestive tracts.

Killing the good bacteria that once resided in my gut with those multiple rounds of antibiotics meant that I needed to rebuild the good bacteria in my gut. **My first "tool" in my "healing" tool kit was a strong probiotic** that I ingested first thing every morning on an empty stomach, so it could get the probiotics into my *empty* gut and begin to restore and repair it. According to Harvard Medical Review,

> "...probiotics may be of use in aiding urogenital (vaginal) health...and restores balance of common female urogenital problems...[such] as urinary tract infection."[10]

A probiotic complex is an important jump-start to your bladder's healing because, according to the Mayo Clinic,

> "Probiotics may prevent and treat urinary tract infections as well as offer protection from harmful bacteria."[11]

In addition, there is some evidence that athletes who took probiotic supplements suffered fewer symptoms of illness and recovered sooner than those who did not.

There are several probiotic complexes on the market; I have used Swanson Ultra Veggie Capsules[12] which contain Lactobacillus rhamnosus/two billion viable organisms; Lactobacillus acidophilus/1 billion viable organisms; Lactococcus lactis/500 million viable organisms;

Bifidobacterium longum/500 million viable organisms; Streptococcus thermophilus/200 million viable organisms; and FOS (fructooligosaccharides), 400 milligrams.

You might also try Bio-acidophilus Forte[13] available on the Internet from revital [sic]. One bottle contains 30 capsules to be taken one per day, and each capsule contains a staggering 30 billion viable cells of the unique LAB4 complex of probiotic cells. Gregor Reid of the Lawson Health Research Institute has said,

> "...there have been no documented cases of probiotic overdose."[14]

It appears that if you take too much of a probiotic supplement, your body gets rid of the excess bacteria through fecal waste.

The second tool in my IC arsenal is Vitamin C with protective bioflavonoids, Acerola and Wild Rose Hips (1000 milligrams Vitamin C as ascorbic acid; Citrus Bioflavonoid Complex 50 milligrams; Acerola extract 50 milligrams; Rose Hips 10 milligrams). This is available commercially at Puritan's Pride.[15] Take 1000 milligrams of Vitamin C daily (in one dose or as two 500 milligrams doses taken separately; one in the morning and one in the evening).

Vitamin C is a powerful, natural, antibiotic-type supplement that helps ward off many types of diseases and "body bugs." Because of its antibiotic-type properties, it is *the* main ingredient in cold remedies such as Emergen-C and Airborne. These products help fortify our bodies against free radical attacks. Airborne is marketed to help us as we breathe

the same contaminated air over and over again during airline flights. Emergen-C is marketed to help boost our immune system. Both of these products work to fortify our immune system with mega-doses of Vitamin C. This makes sense since Vitamin C is a natural anti-microbial, anti-bacterial supplement.

Vitamin C creates a hostile environment within the body, and therefore reduces the opportunity for bacterial growth in the bladder. UTIs, in a nutshell, result from bacterial growth in the bladder. One thousand milligrams of Vitamin C daily will help maintain a hostile environment in your bladder to minimize opportunities for bacterial growth.

Too much Vitamin C results in diarrhea so, if you develop loose or watery stools, reduce your dose until your stools become formed again. Be assured, you will certainly recognize when you have ingested enough or too much Vitamin C into your system.

The third tool in the IC tool kit is a cranberry fruit concentrate. I take Puritan's Pride Cranberry Fruit Concentrate [this is a supplement. *Not* to be confused with fruit juice concentrate!] 4200 milligrams.[16]

Many urologists believe that cranberry supplements, because they are highly concentrated, when taken in conjunction with Vitamin C, complete the establishment of a hostile environment within the bladder to control bacterial growth. The level of concentration needed to establish that environment *cannot* be obtained from cranberry juice.

Further, cranberry juice—due to its high oxalate content—can lead to the development of kidney stones.[17]

Only physicians from the dinosaur era would recommend cranberry juice today for a UTI or for IC sufferers. This is because juice has an extremely high sugar content and sugar fuels bacterial growth in the bladder (that is the underlying reason we are counseled to drink lots of water when we have a UTI or IC flare). Therefore, *always avoid cranberry juice!* Our bodies convert sugar and sugary drinks and candies into acid. Acid is bad for IC/UTI sufferers. It is the sugar (a known bladder irritant) that quickly sends the body's pH balance to the highly acidic side of the pH spectrum. One reason it can burn to urinate is because the urine in our body has become acidic. Choose cranberry supplements, taken in conjunction with Vitamin C, instead of cranberry juice … you'll be glad you did.

Burning urine was the reason I searched for and used the fourth tool in my tool kit, multiple times every day. **The fourth tool is an alkalizing tea**, or *was* an alkalizing tea; since conducting final edits on this book, I discovered Swanson discontinued this fabulous tea. Yet, it was one of the most wonderful beverages on the planet. It enabled me to finally re-integrate a highly watered-down cup of coffee into my morning fluid intake. While Swanson has discontinued its alkalizing tea, they now offer pH Protector Drops[18] that, added to water or other liquids, help you maintain a proper pH level (look at endnote 18 for more information). Alkalizing tea (or the pH Protector Drops) was the key to maintaining a healthy body pH.

I also drank this tea to alkaline my body when it felt too acidic. I began my day by drinking about eight ounces of water right out of bed, then I drank a cup of alkalizing tea, followed by a cup of watered-down coffee, and then I finished with a second cup of the alkalizing tea (using the tea bag from the first cup over again). In the evening, I occasionally enjoyed a glass of red wine (yes, wine!) with dinner, thanks to Swanson pH Balance Alkalizing Tea. You can use Swanson pH Protector Drops to reduce your body's pH just as I used the alkalizing tea.

I found the water and the two cups of the tea (one before and one after the diluted coffee) were alkalizing enough to partially neutralize the coffee-created acid in my bladder, while also providing enough liquid to flush everything out pretty quickly.

In that most people who suffer with IC tend to have a highly acidic body pH, it became a priority for me to stabilize, restore, and maintain the pH in my body to an alkaline state.

It is my belief that healing is optimized when the body's pH is balanced, and that maintaining a well-balanced pH level is one of the most pivotal things you can do to avoid bladder flares. I have been unable to locate scientific evidence to support my belief, but it seems to me that if an acidic environment makes the bladder feel worse—and possibly lengthens the time it takes to heal bladder ulcers—then an alkaline environment might make the bladder feel better and heal faster.

To check my body's pH, I use EnzyMedica's pH Urine Strips.[19] EnzyMedica pH Urine Strips are available over the counter at most pharmacies, specialty grocers like Sprouts, Vitamin Cottage or Whole Foods and herbal stores. I have found that, over time, I can guesstimate with uncanny accuracy, my body's pH by tuning in to how my bladder feels.

"Health is better than wealth." – English Proverb

Chapter 4

My Expanded Tool Kit - Additional Dietary Supplement Tools

Because I had fabulous success with the previous tools in *My Basic "Healing" Tool Kit*, I decided to delve deeper into dietary supplements that could heal other aspects of my debilitating IC and improve my overall health. This chapter includes information about additional supplements I take, the amounts taken, safety information, some interactions, as well as additional information.

You may find the information in this chapter helpful regarding what parts of the body these supplements may improve or heal, as well as important precaution. When noted, be sure to access the URL information from the endnotes section for additional important supplement information or go to my website: www.drtracyalexis.com to learn more about the endnotes section of this book.

To get right to these additional supplements, let's begin with an herbal blend that addresses all issues related to the female reproductive system, which includes the bladder, ovaries, and uterus. I call it the "female reproductive" herbal blend and it is a blend of the following herbs: Punarnava (.36 lb), Shatavari (.18 lb), and Gokshura (.36 lb). The herbalist blends these herbs together with the quantities indicated above. I consumed the blended herbs, which were a powder, by mixing ¼ teaspoon of the herbal blend with ¼ cup of fat free milk.

The powder tends to clump in the milk, but the clumps are easily dissolved by gently pressing the clumps against the rim of the cup with a spoon and stirring into the milk. Drink quickly before the herbs settle to the bottom of the cup. Once accustomed to the unusual taste of the herbal blend (it took me about a week), I increased my intake to ½ tsp herbal blend with ¼ cup of fat-free milk (or use an appropriate fat-free milk-substitute of your choice). This herbal blend should be available from any retailer that specializes in (local and imported) herbs. This herbal blend was bought from The Herb Store[20] in Albuquerque, New Mexico.

Calcium

Calcium,[21] in particular, is very alkaline, and it helps restore, promote, and retain a higher body (alkaline) level of pH. All women, young as well as old, need calcium (and Vitamin D, as calcium cannot be absorbed without vitamin D to carry it through the body's metabolic processes) to ensure bone density. Especially as women age, calcium is needed to minimize osteoporosis. If the calcium comes as a "citrate," the citrate[22] combination simply enables the body to absorb the calcium without food and helps move the supplement to the cellular level.

Swanson Vitamin markets a calcium product that addresses the calcium citrate *and* the Vitamin D needs of most women. It is always advisable to check with your health care professional for routine blood panel studies prior to beginning any supplement regime and, after an agreed-upon period of time on that regime, to monitor your blood levels and ensure you are taking only the supplements *you* need.

Swanson Vitamin Calcium Citrate (630 milligrams) and Vitamin D (400 IU)[23] play an important role in preventing chronic pain and in boosting the immune system. Studies have revealed that women with higher levels of Vitamin D had lower levels of pelvic floor disorders[24]—among which IC is included.

Supplement needs vary widely from one individual to the next depending on lifestyle, diet, exercise, and other factors. Be safe and smart in caring for your body by involving your health care professional in your plans to begin taking supplements!

Calcium and Vitamin D overdose symptoms can include loss of appetite; dizziness; nausea; vomiting; mental or mood changes; headache; drowsiness; weakness; tiredness; or trouble breathing. Residents of the United States should call poison control at 1-800-222-1222 for assistance with calcium overdose.

D-3

Vitamin D-3,[25] Cholecalciferol, is marketed by Swanson in 1000 IU strength. While Vitamin D is most commonly used by our bodies to help us absorb calcium and improve bone strength, it is the calcium—which is very alkaline—that is believed to "calm the fire" in urine that most people who suffer from IC experience.

Too much D-3 can lead to high calcium levels, or hypercalcemia, with poor appetite, nausea, and vomiting. Weakness and frequent urination are also possible. Some health care providers have said that calcium toxicity can lead to kidney stones.[26]

In nature, exposure to the sun is what provides D-3 to our bodies. Given the many warnings about harmful UVB ray exposure and the potential for skin cancers from sun-damaged skin, many individuals have decided to take a supplement and avoid the health risks associated with sun exposure.

Vitamin E

Vitamin E[27] as d-alpha Tocopherol Acetate 6 IU. Puritan's Pride taken two times daily. Vitamin E supports red blood cells and helps boost the immune system. My logic indicated that if Vitamin E helped my red blood cells in any way (because red blood cells carry all the nutrients that heal everything that is situated deep within our bodies, like the bladder), I want my blood to be the very best it can be.

If undergoing surgery, stop taking Vitamin E at least two weeks beforehand. Because Vitamin E and other antioxidant vitamins (Vitamin C and beta carotene) seem to interfere with the healing process, one should avoid taking them immediately before or after surgery outside the supervision of a health care professional. Also, there is a LOT of additional information regarding Vitamin E contained within the footnotes at the end of this book. Please be sure to check those web addresses, as well as ask your primary care physician, for important information before incorporating Vitamin E into your daily supplement intake.

Swanson markets natural Vitamin E as d-alpha Tocopherol acetate[28] and I took 20 IU. "Vitamin E" actually refers to a group of eight different compounds that work to build a healthy immune system, skin, hair, and nails.[29] Some say that Vitamin E increases endurance, improves energy, reduces muscle damage after exercise, and increases muscle strength, but there are dangers.

Vitamin E is possibly unsafe if taken by mouth in high doses. If you have a condition such as heart disease or diabetes, you should not take doses of 400 IU per day or higher. Some research suggests that high doses might increase the chances of other serious side effects or even death. The higher the dose you take, of course, the higher the risks.

There is some concern that Vitamin E might increase the chance of having a hemorrhagic stroke (bleeding in the brain). Some research suggests that Vitamin E in doses of 300-800 IU daily might increase the chances of such a stroke by as much as 22%. However, in contrast, Vitamin E might *decrease* the chances of the less severe ischemic stroke.

Information about the effect of Vitamin E on the development of prostate cancer is contradictory. Some research suggests that taking large amounts of a multivitamin plus a separate Vitamin E supplement might increase the risk of prostate cancer in some men. High doses can also cause nausea, diarrhea, stomach cramps, fatigue, weakness, headache, blurred vision, rash, bruising, and bleeding. In people with a history of cancer, Vitamin E supplements in doses of 400 IU or more could increase the probability that their cancer will return. There is also concern that Vitamin E might increase the risk of developing prostate cancer. The effect of Vitamin E on existing prostate cancer is not clear. However, it is possible that Vitamin E could worsen it.

When used in the recommended daily amount, Vitamin E is *possibly safe* for pregnant women. There has been some concern that taking Vitamin E supplements might be harmful to the fetus during early pregnancy. However, it is too soon to say with any certainty. Until more is known, Vitamin E supplements should *not* be taken during early pregnancy unless your physician approves.

Vitamin E is *likely safe* when taken by mouth in the recommended daily amounts during breast- feeding. Vitamin E is also *likely safe* when taken by mouth appropriately by infants and children. The maximum amounts are based on age: less than 200 milligrams daily for children 1 to 3 years old; less than 300 milligrams daily is safe for children 4 to 8 years old; less than 600 milligrams daily is safe for children 9 to 13 years old; and less than 800 milligrams daily is considered safe for children 14 to 18 years old. Vitamin E is *possibly unsafe* when given intravenously in high doses to premature infants.

Vitamin E might increase the risk of heart failure in people with diabetes and so they should avoid high doses. In high doses Vitamin E also might increase the risk of death in people with a history of heart attack. Those with a history of stroke as well as people with blood clotting problems, especially those with low levels of Vitamin K, should also avoid high doses of Vitamin E. A dose of 400 IU of *synthetic* Vitamin E seems to speed vision loss in people with retinitis pigmentosa but much lower amounts (e.g., 3 IU) do not seem to have this effect. Nevertheless, people with retinitis pigmentosa should probably avoid Vitamin E supplements. Likewise, people with bleeding disorders should avoid taking Vitamin E.

Iodine

Iodine[30] (liquid iodine with potassium iodide) 3 drops taken daily (generally mixed with water). This product is manufactured by Life-flo and available from Swanson Vitamins.[31] Aside from the benefits to our thyroid, iodine is a vitally important nutrient found in every organ and tissue in the body. It is essential to healthy metabolism—the process that stokes the body and turns ingested food into fuel, burning it off as it is used or collecting it into fat cells if it is not. The key to a healthy weight is our metabolism and how our bodies turn food into fuel and iodine is extremely important for a healthy metabolism.

Oral ingestion of iodine can cause severe damage to the mouth, esophagus, and lungs, and it may result in shortness of breath, edema of the glottis (a vocal component of the larynx), or pulmonary edema (fluid accumulation in the lungs). Vomiting, abdominal pain, diarrhea, and severe gastroenteritis may also follow oral ingestion as well as a metallic taste in the mouth and possible renal failure. Shock is also possible, which can result in an increased heart rate, low blood pressure, and a complete collapse of the circulatory system. Oral ingestion of iodine can also affect the brain, causing headache, dizziness, and delirium. As such, I strongly recommend consulting your health care provider before adding an iodine supplement to your diet.

Quercetin Bromelain

Swanson Quercetin Bromelain[32] (Quercetin from Sophora japonica flower buds [500 milligrams]; Bromelain from pineapple [156 milligrams]). Quercetin is a flavonoid, a group of plant (polyphenolic) metabolites thought to provide health benefits that are found in fresh vegetables and fruits. While many benefits are assured, Quercetin, like everything on the market today, is accompanied by risks.

I am confident that I have felt much better while taking Quercetin Bromelain although only two medical studies have been conducted on the specific effects of it on people with IC. According to the University of Maryland Medical Center, fewer symptoms were experienced by test participants when taking Quercetin but other flavonoids with properties comparable to Quercetin were in the substances given to the test subjects.[33] This means that patients who have *any* type of medical condition, especially cancer, should check with their physicians or oncologist prior to taking Quercetin.

Little is known about the effects of an overdose of Quercetin.[34] It is not even clear if an overdose is possible or how much Quercetin could cause an overdose. If you think you have overdosed on any supplement, you must seek medical attention immediately!

Research on Bromelain is in its infancy, but it is believed to reduce swelling, pain, bruising, and to reduce recovery time following surgery or traumatic injuries. Some societies use Bromelain to treat inflammation and indigestion because of its protein-digesting enzymes. It has also been used to remove dead tissue surrounding second- and third-degree burns, to treat inflammation from insect stings and bites, and it has reportedly been used to treat symptoms of hay fever.

We do not know what to expect from a Bromelain overdose or, indeed, if such an overdose is possible. It might be that an overdose could increase the risk of bleeding, including internal bleeding, but this is still in the hypothetical stage.

As mentioned elsewhere in this book, many professional health care providers know very little about topics outside their specialties. You should ask specifically whether your health care provider is knowledgeable about dietary supplements beyond his/her medical expertise. Ask him or her how long they have worked with individuals on non-traditional or holistic interventions. How long and how often have they prescribed supplements instead of medications or synthetics (man-made chemicals) for healing, and how long have they prescribed non-traditional health remedies or alternatives? Ask if they have case studies of their successes they can share. Ask whether they self-supplement? Ask! Ask! Ask!

Any questions you think are important to your understanding regarding the strengths your health care provider can offer you are questions you want and need to have answered! In this way you can ensure that your questions about supplements and/or medications are being answered by someone with knowledge, experience, and some level of expertise. By knowing with confidence that your health care provider is informed and offering known recommendations, you can have peace of mind about their suggestions and move forward to live a happy, healthy, productive life.

MSM

MSM[35] (methyl-sulfonyl-methane) is the third largest ingredient in the human body and found in all vertebrates. Touted by some as the miracle supplement, MSM is a chemically inert (inactive) organic sulfur compound derived naturally from the earth's rain cycle. MSM is said to increase energy, heal the body, provide anti-inflammatory benefits, strengthen hair and nails, improve flexibility, detoxify the body, and improve skin and complexion.[36] It helps the body produce its own antioxidants (found naturally in fruits and vegetables)—that is, MSM retards oxidation which is a chain reaction that can lead to cell damage. Common side effects of overdose[37] are gastrointestinal discomfort, nausea, vomiting, diarrhea, and cramps.

Turmeric

Turmeric[38] (Curcuma longa), a rhizome, is also marketed by Swanson Vitamins. Used for more than 5000 years, it is appreciated mostly for its anti-inflammatory (which helps eliminate pain), anti-microbial (which kills the microbes that cause acne, and other germs), and detoxification properties. It can also boost the immune system and, with at least one disease, modulate the immune response. It might also be safe when used in the short-term as an enema or as a mouthwash.

Turmeric usually does not have significant side effects. However, some people can experience stomach upset, nausea, dizziness, or diarrhea. In one report, a person who took very high amounts of turmeric (over 1500 milligrams twice daily) experienced a dangerously abnormal heart rhythm.[39] However, it is unclear whether turmeric was the actual cause of this reaction. In the meantime, play it safe and avoid taking excessively high doses. High amounts of turmeric might also prevent the absorption of iron. It also might slow blood clotting and therefore bleeding both during and after surgery. I recommend you stop ingesting turmeric at least two weeks before a scheduled surgery.

With regard to women who are pregnant or who are breast-feeding, turmeric is likely safe when taken in amounts commonly found in food. However, it is likely *unsafe* when taken by mouth in medicinal amounts during pregnancy. Such use might promote a menstrual period or stimulate the uterus thus putting the pregnancy at risk. Since there is not enough information to rate the safety of medicinal amounts of turmeric during breast-feeding, it is safest not to take it at all.

Turmeric can also exacerbate gall bladder problems. Do not use it if you have gallstones or a bile duct obstruction. Turmeric can also cause stomach upset and it might make some problems like GERD[40] worse.

Turmeric might lower testosterone levels and decrease sperm movement in men when taken orally. Turmeric should therefore be used cautiously by couples seeking to get pregnant.

Curcumin, a chemical in turmeric, might decrease blood sugar in people with diabetes. And it might behave like the hormone estrogen. In theory, turmeric might make some hormone-sensitive conditions worse. However, some research has shown that turmeric reduces the effects of estrogen in some hormone-sensitive cancer cells. Until more is known about curcumin, it should be used cautiously if you have a condition that might be made worse by exposure to hormones.

Multi-Mineral Citrate Complex

Swanson Multi-Mineral Citrate Complex[41] is an alkalizing agent (calcium from calcium citrate 75 milligrams;

magnesium from magnesium citrate, 30 milligrams; zinc from zinc citrate 2 milligrams; potassium from potassium citrate[42] 49.5 milligrams) and is, in general, very positive for restoring the body's natural pH balance.

Serious side effects of potassium citrate include uneven heartbeat, muscle weakness or a limp feeling, severe stomach pain, and numbness in the hands, feet, or mouth. However, *do not stop taking this supplement* without first talking to your physician.[43]

Overdose symptoms of calcium citrate might include nausea, vomiting, decreased appetite, constipation, confusion, delirium, stupor, and coma. Magnesium citrate overdoses are not commonly reported but they can include diarrhea and severe stomach pain. If this happens you should call a poison control center immediately.[44]

Zinc

Zinc[45] is one of the 24 micronutrients needed for survival. It is found in meat, eggs, and legumes (be careful of lintels, as they are high in oxalic acid and *not* on the IC-friendly diet). Oysters are a particularly good source of zinc. Marketed by Swanson Vitamins as Zinc Gluconate in 30 milligrams dosages, it is also an aphrodisiac and a testosterone builder, but it will only elevate testosterone levels if the user is already deficient in zinc. Zinc is also very important for enzyme, hormone, and immune system functioning systems but it is lost through perspiration, which means it should be replenished with supplemental intake—this is important for athletes who may not get enough zinc through their normal food intake.

Gotu Kola

I also incorporated an herb called Gotu Kola[46] (aerial parts), which retails from Swanson Vitamins in a 435-milligram dose, and which has also been used as an alternative to medication for treating venous insufficiency (decreased blood flow). Again, my desire was for my blood and the veins carrying my blood to various parts of my body—including and especially the deepest tissues, muscles, organs, etc.—be the healthiest it could be so as to improve any deficits in my blood and its flow, with the overarching goal of healing my body's insides.

Vitamin A

Vitamin A, also known as Beta Carotene[47] is marketed by Swanson Vitamins in a 10,000 IU dose and is an essential nutrient (see next paragraph). Beta carotene promotes healthy skin and mucus membranes. Since membrane-like tissue comprises the bladder, I decided to incorporate Vitamin A, which is an essential vitamin, into my supplement intake. Beta carotene is converted to Vitamin A and, if added through our food intake, our bodies convert only the amount of Vitamin A that is needed. Importantly, supplement intake of Vitamin A can result in toxicity if taken at high levels.

An *essential* nutrient is a nutrient required for normal body functioning, but which cannot be produced by the body.[48]

Vitamin B and other B-complexes

Vitamin B[49] is an important supplement because it is key in developing blood cells, converting food into energy for the body, preventing anemia, and facilitating the body's enzyme reaction to amino acids (amino acids are building blocks for the body's immune system and will be discussed later in the book). Taking a Vitamin B complex is also instrumental in regulating sleep, mood, and in maintaining brain function and cell metabolism. Healthy cell metabolism permits the replacement of damaged cells in the bladder as the body constantly renews its cellular structure, strengthening and fortifying the bladder lining over time.

In general, a Vitamin B overdose can lead to heart failure or kidney problems, including kidney failure. Because there are so many different B vitamins, here is a very condensed list of health problems that could result from ingesting too much of the listed B vitamin. Of course, you should always consult your physician to ensure that the supplement you want to take is appropriate for your medical needs and/or for your desired health outcome.

Vitamin B1   Skin rashes; allergic reactions; agitation; insomnia; heart palpitations

Vitamin B2   Fatigue; vomiting; nausea; hypotension; dark yellowish urine

Vitamin B3	Headache; skin rash; flushing; joint pain; nausea; vomiting; insomnia
Vitamin B6	Numbness in the extremities; tingling sensations; muscle cramps; restlessness; fatigue; mood swings; and insomnia
Vitamin B9	Bloating; anorexia or decrease in appetite
Vitamin B12	Tingling sensation; panic attacks; insomnia; heart palpitations

All Day Energy Greens

When I was diagnosed with Interstitial Cystitis, I began my research on how to rebuild my body's immune system from the inside. My rationale was that, since my problem (IC) was *inside* my body, I needed to repair the *inside* of my body!

Fruits and vegetables are the building blocks of healthy cells which, in turn, build healthy tissues, and healthy tissue was my focus in order to repair my damaged bladder. I began drinking All Day Energy Greens[50]—a highly concentrated powder with one scoop being equivalent to five servings of fruits and vegetables. I now drink at least one 8-ounce serving of this beverage every day. It mixes well with water and has a pleasant taste. When I first began drinking this, I mixed my Energy Greens with Guava juice, then quickly switched to water when I learned of the juice's high sugar content.

Within two years, my appetite increased, as did my bladder capacity, which went from less than an ounce of capacity after my bladder's death and painful function restoration to hold approximately eight ounces before I needed to void. After four years of drinking All Day Energy Greens daily, my bladder capacity has increased to about 14 ounces, give or take—this is a miraculous turn-around coming from my total bladder death! I find my 14-ounce bladder capacity today is a medically remarkable increase, which I take to mean that my body is healing nicely!

Superfoods/Antioxidants/Anti-inflammatory

I also added to my diet alfalfa,[51] green barley,[52] spirulina,[53] kelp,[54] chlorella,[55] wheat grass,[56] chlorophyll,[57] and blue-green algae[58] as supplemental "superfood" greens,[59] with phenomenal results. These dietary Superfoods[60] are available at most health food stores (like Sprouts or Whole Foods, etc.). Also available as a dietary supplement is Co-Q-10[61] taken in 30-60 milligram doses; it is the "queen of the antioxidants." I also take Omega 3 fats, such as Salmon Oil[62] and RxOmega-3,[63] Pharmaceutical Grade Fish Oil (EPA400 milligrams/DHA 200 milligrams), which help keep the heart and circulatory system working at maximum efficiency.[64] Ground flaxseed (which also contains Omega 3 fats) was, and continues to be, added to meatloaf (in place of bread crumbs) and to my breakfast oatmeal and smoothies.

Lastly, because I have always genuinely enjoyed spicy foods (but IC sufferers are strongly cautioned to avoid spicy foods due to their highly acidic content), I learned that cayenne pepper[65] contains amazing anti-inflammatory properties, while also provides a little "heat" to foods without the accompanying adverse side effects of acidic spices! If you question this, I invite you to prove it for yourself: The next time you have a sore throat, mix a cup of hot water with a squeeze of fresh lemon, add a dollop of honey and a 1/8 teaspoon of cayenne pepper, and drink it. The beverage will coat your throat and remove the discomfort (but there will be heat on your throat first from the cayenne pepper, then relief from the anti-inflammatory properties which immediately remove that previous throat discomfort). And, when this beverage comes out (the other end), it does *not* burn!

Teas

In addition to the Alkalizing Tea referenced in Chapter 3, I also enjoyed two or three cups of Agaricus XP Mushroom Tea[66] (available from Noevir) for the first two months following my IC diagnosis, and then once per day *every day,* after I started feeling better. Mushrooms are very powerful yielding health benefits for cancer, heart health, immunity, diabetes, and weight management.[67]

Other teas you may consider that are IC-friendly are: (a) corn silk;[68] (b) marshmallow root;[69] and (c) horsetail.[70] These teas are available "loose."

ASEA

ASEA[71] liquid, which initially tastes like pool water and is pH balanced to our body's natural pH level, should be taken two to three times per day to help soothe the bladder from the inside. ASEA Redox, is the world's first and only stabilized balanced redox cell signaling supplement. It is the native molecules that cause our cells to recognize abnormal cells and kill them off (apoptosis), recognize damage and repair it, regenerate cells and turn on normal gene expression. We produce these tiny molecules in high abundance as children and less and less as we age or are exposed to poor diet, lack of exercise, medications and diseases, including IC and fibromyalgia.

ASEA Redox commonly tastes like swimming pool water when you first drink it. After a limited period of detoxification, the pool water taste goes away and there is no taste. A dosage of 6-8 ounces in two to three divided doses, not mixed with anything else ingested at least five minutes before or 20 minutes after eating is recommended to help reduce inflammation and swelling from the inside.

ASEA mimics the chemical composition of normal saline and can also be used as a soothing *instillation*—instilled directly into the bladder through a catheter—to help calm a fiery bladder. Of course, you will need to become proficient with self-catheterization as well as with the appropriate sterile techniques to perform an ASEA instillation (read about how to master self-catheterization in Chapter 6).

There are internet critics who claim ASEA Redox is just expensive salt water,[72] but my experiences were very powerfully positive, especially using ASEA Redox as an instillation. Extensive studies have shown there is absolutely no toxicity with the human identical molecules in ASEA

Redox and ASEA Redox does not interact with drugs supplements or herbs.[73]

Natural (Rock or Sea) Salt

Replace your iodized (synthetic; man-made) table salt with a natural salt that contains trace minerals![74] Natural salt will *not* have iodine as an ingredient, so if you have a medical condition that requires you to take iodine; you should consult with your physician before you follow this recommendation. Otherwise, if iodine is not medically necessary for you, you may opt to take trace mineral drops.

Minerals

The following combination of mineral supplements helps promote cardiovascular health, promotes relaxation, and works wonders for the circulatory system: Solaray Magnesium and Potassium Asporotates,[75] which is comprised of Magnesium 300 milligrams, Potassium 40 milligrams and Bromelain 140 milligrams. The medical community does not yet know exactly how this combination of supplements provide their benefits, but the following information on each one taken by itself might shed more light.

Magnesium is a vitally important supplement for cardiovascular health and immune function. It fortifies our nerves and muscles and it also keeps bones strong, regulates heart rhythm, and regulates blood sugars and blood pressure. It is also a key component in protein synthesis. Halibut, nuts, beans, and spinach are great sources of magnesium, but note that spinach is *not* on the IC diet because of its high oxalic acid content (which is strongly suspected to trigger IC flares).

Dietary magnesium does not pose a health risk. However, pharmacological doses of magnesium in supplements can produce adverse effects such as diarrhea and abdominal cramping when taken in excess.

Potassium is also an essential mineral for the body. It is an electrolyte mineral that (because it is metal) helps conduct electricity, making it essential for healthy heart function and smooth muscle contraction. Evidence suggests that a diet rich in potassium promotes bone health and can lower the risk of stroke. Avocados, lima beans, flounder, salmon, cod, and chicken are all rich in potassium and are all on the IC diet.

Symptoms of hyperkalemia, or too much potassium, include irregular heartbeat, nausea, and slow, weak, or even absent pulse.

Bromelain is discussed in previous pages of this book with additional information under Endnotes 32 and 33. However, as a enzyme found in pineapple, Bromelain is beneficial medically for reducing swelling, among other things. Lastly, Bromelain can also be obtained from mangoes, honey, papaya, bananas, avocados and kefir, which are gentle foods for IC sufferers. As indicated at the beginning of this paragraph, bromelain is also found in pineapple, although pineapple is a highly acidic fruit and can exacerbate IC discomfort and create "burning" urine.

AMINO ACIDS

There are about 500 amino acids[76] within the human body. These are complex, biologically significant, body-building components, and the protein form of amino acids helps compose the body's cells and tissues, including muscles. Other categories of amino acids regulate the pH (acid/alkaline balance) within the body. As such, amino acids are central to not only healing damaged tissues but also for providing the body's environmental climate to manifest miraculous results.

In addition to branched-chain amino acids (referenced and discussed below), my research revealed two specific amino acids to target the results I wanted for my bladder healing (L-Lysine and L-Arginine).

L-Lysine

L-Lysine[77] is one of the two such amino acid building blocks, and 500 milligrams taken one to two times daily is very important. However, large doses of L-Lysine can cause diarrhea and stomach cramps. Our bodies need this building block, but we cannot manufacture it internally, so it should be taken only as directed on the supplement label, and then only after you have discussed its intake with your health care provider.

Essential amino acids are *not* created by or stored in our bodies (like fat is stored in our body's fat cells) so the foods we eat must provide us with these important building blocks on a constant, continuous basis. Swanson Vitamins markets

L-Lysine (from AJI Pure Pharmaceutical Grade L-Lysine HCI) in 500 milligram doses.[78]

Typically, meats, dairy, legumes, and grains provide our bodies with the requisite quantities of L-Lysine.

Tillery, et al., writing in <u>Integrated Science</u>[79] (2001), have said that some popular ethnic foods can provide all ten amino acids: Cajun red beans and rice, Mexican corn and beans, and Japanese rice and soybeans. In general, a Lysine overdose is not considered to be life-threatening and the symptoms, if any, are mild.

L-Arginine

L-Arginine,[80] a free-form amino acid, is marketed by Swanson Vitamins in 500 milligram doses.[81] This supplement is said to increase blood flow and help relax bladder muscle spasms so it might, thereby, help control IC pain. The body converts L-Arginine into nitric oxide, which opens blood vessels widely and also stimulates the release of growth hormones. As I have noted elsewhere in this book, as a building block of the body's immune system, L-Arginine helps the body heal both inside (as with IC) and outside (as with a cut, scrape, or burn on the skin).

Once again, it is important to consult with your health care provider before beginning a regimen that includes L-Arginine. Nausea, vomiting, diarrhea, worsening of asthma or allergies, and hypotension are all possible side effects of excess L-Arginine in the bloodstream but little information is currently available.

As you can probably determine, I spent significant amounts of money for the above supplements, teas, antioxidants, etc., but then, I considered my health to be well worth the investment it took to get my body healed. For me, this was a very serious commitment ... a commitment worth making, but I am sharing this because if you are not committed to creating a healthy body and resulting good health, then justifying the expense could provide a tremendous physical, emotional, and financial challenge. These are decisions each reader must reach on her/his own.

Branched Chain Amino Acids (BCAA)

There are 20 different amino acids that make up the thousands of different proteins in the human body.[82] Nine of those 20 are considered essential, which means our body cannot produce them and they must, therefore, be obtained through the foods we eat. Of those nine amino acids, three are the branched chain amino acids (BCAA). These branched chain amino acids are: leucine, isoleucine and valine. Branched chain basically refers to the chemical structure of the BCAAs, which are found in protein-rich foods such as dairy, meat and eggs. In a nutshell, amino acids are the building blocks of a healthy body.

There are numerous benefits of including branched chain amino acids in our diets. For those BCAAs our bodies cannot produce, it benefits us to take a supplement. BCAAs are beneficial for building muscles, decreasing muscle soreness, reducing fatigue from exercise, preventing muscle wasting, and helping people who have liver disease.[83]

I take a supplement called Amino Complete[84]- because it contains ALL of the amino acids as well as vitamin B-6.

DIET

Because the foods we eat pass through our bodies and nourish (or damage) it, I made another commitment to put the best foods I could possibly afford into my damaged body. It was strongly recommended that I avoid all processed and preservative-laden foods. To ensure that I was not voluntarily adding harmful chemicals into my body, I decided to purchase organic foods whenever organic was available. While organic foods *do* cost more, the health results are far-reaching and my excellent health is worth this additional financial investment.

The women's urology specialist suggested a strict, exceptionally low-acid diet that I call the *white diet*. If it is white, and thus bland and typically less nutritious with no taste-bud excitement, then I can eat it—and you can, too!

There are dietary specialists who say that white foods are what one should *not* eat: white bread, white rice, white potatoes, white sugar, etc. I don't eat white bread because it is the standard from which the glycemic index is derived (and I am hypoglycemic) and so, from that point of view, no diet could be worse for me. White potatoes—and those include the little red-skinned ones that are white on the inside—also have a high glycemic index, as does white rice.

I don't eat white rice because our bodies convert white rice into sugar, and sugar is the IC sufferers' number one enemy. You, too, may need to start with a white (or *bland*) diet and gradually move toward foods that are more to your liking, as I did. But we all must begin somewhere when our bladder function is compromised, and the white/bland diet is where I began.

I also began keeping a diary of my food intake for each meal and in-between-meal snacks, so that if I experienced physical discomfort, I could trace my physical discomfort back to the food source. The daily diary has proved itself a remarkable tool over and over again, helping me eliminate certain foods completely from my intake! You will locate a useable daily diary template in the appendix section of this book.

After about eight months of bland foods, I was permitted to *gradually* add more tasteful foods to my food intake. I monitored everything I consumed by entering those foods into my daily diary and noted that sugary foods resulted in urine that burned coming out when I had to void. Again, I learned that sugar creates an acidic, bacteria-friendly environment within the bladder, which I wanted to avoid.

It is important that you understand how sugar affects the bladder because a diet heavy in sugar unfortunately leads to IC flare-ups. Flare-ups (or *flares* as most IC sufferers refer to them) mimic a urinary tract infection, but flares lack the accompanying bacterial growth that requires taking a round of antibiotics. An IC flare tricks you into believing you have a UTI because of the resulting burning, highly uncomfortable, and frequent urination.

Trust me when I share that to keep flares—and UTIs—to a minimum, you must avoid sugar and processed foods, like pasta, corn, potatoes, breads, white flour, cakes and cookies, that convert to sugar during the body's metabolic process; all of these foods are converted to sugar through our body's metabolic process, and thus, all of these foods turn our body's pH acidic. Since sugar is one of the main ingredients in so many processed foods, you need to become very attentive and resolute in your efforts to avoid sugar. It may feel difficult because sugar is added to almost every processed food available in the United States. You CAN and MUST eliminate sugar from your diet!

Eliminating or significantly reducing sugar requires practice and persistence by: (1) reading labels; (2) getting familiar with the foods that contain sugars; (3) making a commitment to avoid those foods; and (4) adjusting your taste to less-sweet foods/products. Focused determination to restore your body to a healthy pH balance will benefit your overall well-being and, more importantly, will jump-start your bladder's healing.

Instead of sugar, I use stevia, which is a natural, plant-based sweetener. Because of my sensitivity to chemicals, I spend the extra money and purchase organic stevia whenever it is available. There is also a product called monk fruit that can offer sweetness to your diet without the ill effects of refined sugars. Both stevia and monk fruit are available in stores that cater to healthy eating.

The next major key to healing your bladder is to avoid processed foods. The more processed a food, the less nutrition it offers your body. Period.

A good example to consider when determining how much or how little a food has been processed is this: A whole roasted chicken is less processed than a chicken that has been cut into pieces, e.g., the drumsticks, breasts, thighs, etc. Of the two choices, the whole chicken will be healthier. In the United States, with almost every processing step a chicken undergoes—from capture to slaughter to preparation for the consumer—precautionary steps are taken to minimize contamination. Sometimes these precautionary steps are in the form of chemicals which will agitate sensitive bladders and IC. Did you know that each and every time a chicken is cut into smaller pieces it goes through a wash or bath of chemicals to ensure the chicken has no contaminants as it moves forward to its next step in the processing line?

When the chicken pieces undergo further processing—called *secondary* processing—to make strips, nuggets, etc., the real IC irritants are added: nitrates and nitrites (which are toxic food preservatives sometimes referred to as *sodium* nitrate or *sodium* nitrite). These are typically found in all processed meats like sausage, bacon, pre-packaged and deli meats, and many wines also contain nitrites—just read the label on the bottle or packages. It is important that those diagnosed with IC avoid foods containing nitrates and nitrites!

Sometimes hormones and antibiotics are added to chicken (and other processed meats); however, Walmart stocks antibiotic- and hormone-free, boneless, and skinless chicken breasts in individually sealed five-packs (meaning, five breasts, each in its own smaller packaging) under its specialty brand Marketside at a very affordable price. Walmart also carries deli turkey breast that is nitrate- and nitrite-free. Once again, just read the labels on the packages. And if you live in a rural area without a Walmart or comparable supermarket, advocate with your local grocers to carry some organic foods, and nitrate- and nitrite-free meats, along with good-quality vitamin supplements, and teas (or purchase supplements and teas online and have them shipped to your door).

A word to the wise: While shopping for foods, be aware that pesticides and herbicides are used significantly in today's farming/agriculture industry … and some of these chemicals have been linked to dramatic, unwanted health conditions.[85] As such, many of the "fresh" fruits and vegetables offered for purchase are inherently toxic because of the chemical sprays used to keep bugs and other critters from eating them before they reach the market. Chemicals *on and in* foods should be avoided by IC sufferers, as well as added hormones, antibiotics, nitrites and nitrates that are often contained in processed meats.

Lastly, right after my IC diagnosis and for approximately two years following that diagnosis, intestinal gas (flatulence) was one of my largest pain-producing experiences. It took time for me to figure out what was causing my very sharp, intense, and nearly debilitating abdominal pain. This is where the food chart referenced in the appendix revealed itself to be so helpful, because I would notice that an hour or two after eating one of my favorite dishes—pinto beans—my abdominal pain would become excruciatingly unbearable. It took time to correlate that pain to the pinto bean dish I had recently enjoyed. Nevertheless, I quickly learned that chewable papaya enzymes[86] were much better at eliminating intestinal gas than the commercially marketed anti-gas products.

"Let today be the day you give up who you've been for who you can become." – Hal Elrod

Chapter 5

Exercise

In this short chapter, I want to talk about exercise as an important part of healing Interstitial Cystitis. Our bodies need movement to stimulate blood flow to all our appendages and organs. Blood flow is an important component of the healing process, as it brings nutrient-rich, fresh blood to damaged tissues. The tissues and body's internal infrastructure are what we need to heal when it comes to IC, so getting the blood moving throughout the body is important for carrying oxygen and blood-rich nutrients throughout the body to rebuild it.

With IC, movement must be gentle. Your body is damaged or traumatized, so invigorating exercise could create additional damage. The last thing your body needs as you are working to heal it is strenuous, vigorous exercise. Gentle stretching exercises like Pilates, yoga or Tai-chi are excellent for gently stretching the body and moving blood to its extremities. I loved Tai-chi, a martial art form that I found to be very soothing and relaxing, which our local community center offered for free (with a suggested "tip" for the instructor's time to facilitate the free classes).

After the first year of gentle movement exercises, I was able to progress to more stimulating exercise like walking at a constant pace between 30 minutes to an hour each day. Likewise, deep breathing exercise helps increase blood flow, elevates heart rate, and lowers blood pressure. Try the "Breath of Fire"[87] (comparable to how a dog "pants" for breath), which is a short and rapid breathing component of yoga. Walking while deep breathing (or while integrating the "Breath of Fire") might easily be the most under-rated exercise combination, and yet both are so wonderful for invigorating blood flow. A brisk walk is even better but jogging or running should be avoided, at least initially.

If you have ever spoken to a woman who has "pelvic organ prolapse"[88] (where the uterus, bladder, vaginal walls have become "displaced"), you will understand the important need for doing Kegel[89] exercises. As much as most women despise Kegels, I would much rather do Kegels than have a prolapsed uterus or prolapsed bladder (which means it has fallen out of place, sometimes, especially with the uterus, it can exit the body completely—a horrible situation, indeed). Kegel exercises are extremely important for the body overall, as Kegels help strengthen the body's core muscles – the major muscle groups in the body's core. Typically, women who have pelvic floor (and/or prolapse) issues also have trouble voiding and maintaining a properly situated bladder.

Kegel exercises help strengthen the pelvic floor thus ensuring that the bladder, uterus (provided you have not undergone hysterectomy) and surrounding female tissue walls stay in their proper positions and function optimally. If the bladder is where it is supposed to be and is surrounded by strong muscles, it functions *much* better (including strengthening the important ability to start and stop your urine flow mid-stream—practice this to stave off age-related incontinence in your advanced years of life). Just as with other muscles, if these are not used and exercised, they will atrophy and weaken. You can ensure your bladder remains healthy by performing Kegel exercises while stopped at traffic lights, at your desk, riding on elevators, sitting through your child's school play, reading a book, or just about any time and anywhere you think about doing them.

Kegel exercises begin with a slow and steady tightening of the vaginal muscles. Try to picture your vagina as an elevator and imagine that the tighter you squeeze your vaginal muscles the higher the elevator moves. Try to move the elevator up ten (10) floors by squeezing and holding each level or "floor" on which the elevator stops for at least ten seconds, then move your elevator to the next floor and hold that floor's position for ten seconds. Each "floor" should be held for ten seconds before moving the elevator to the next higher floor.

This topic segues naturally into a very important aspect of the professional *medical* treatment of Interstitial Cystitis: instillations.

"Those who can make you believe absurdities can make you commit atrocities." – Voltaire

Chapter 6

Self-Catheterization

At the specialty uro-gynecology (uro-gyn) clinic of our city's university research hospital, my condition was finally diagnosed as Interstitial Cystitis. Following recommendations for diet and exercise, I was scheduled for a weekly procedure called a bladder "instillation," a treatment I mentioned briefly in Chapter 2. Twice weekly instillations were received during the first month; then weekly instillations for the next three months, and then treatments were spaced out less frequently. For months four and five, instillations were spaced two weeks apart; then three weeks apart for two more months; then monthly; and ultimately once per quarter.

I quickly discovered that the quarterly instillations were not frequent enough to keep my bladder functioning at its optimum level so my health care provider and I decided to stay with monthly instillations, and those continued for well over one year. (By the way, I have not received an instillation since 2015!)

The treatment protocol used is as follows (and was "mixed" fresh by the on-site pharmacist literally moments before it was instilled into my bladder through a catheter, *after* any newly produced urine was emptied by the catheter into a collection vessel):

Bupivacaine 0.5% (20 milliliters); Hydrocortisone 100 milligrams (2ML); Heparin 10.000 units (10ML); QS (which means "quantity sufficient" meaning, "add enough of X until the final amount is 60 ML," because, when putting several different ingredients together, it sometimes takes a little more or a little less of X, which is usually saline or water, to reach the final desired amount) with normal saline (20 ML) for a total of 60ML instillation. This mixture was presented in a very large syringe which was subsequently attached to the end of the already-inserted catheter and then slowly pushed from the syringe into my bladder.

The instillation treatment was intended to be held in the bladder for 30 minutes, then flushed out by urinating. I found that the bupivacaine numbed me so well there were several occurrences where I was unable to get the medication out of my body in a 30-minute time-frame (and therefore held the medication until the fullness in my bladder indicated I should release it).

These instillations were extremely soothing!

As part of these treatments, I was educated by the nurse on how to self-catheterize[90] in case I ever experienced another complete bladder shutdown. To me, going through the pain and gyrations of self-catheterization is complete misery.

Correction: When I self-cathed, I was *already* beyond miserable. Self-cathing was done when I could not empty my bladder at the time my body prompted me to. Several times during my healing journey I sat endlessly on the toilet and waited in complete desolation with the sensation of knowing I had to empty my bladder, hoping that even a drop or two would trickle out, and provide some small measure of relief, but nothing would leave my body. If you have experienced similar misery, then I encourage you to learn how to self-cath.

For those of you who have Interstitial Cystitis, you owe it to yourself to learn how to locate your urethra and insert a catheter into it. Develop this skill. You will want to ensure you have the appropriate *sterile* supplies wherever and whenever you might need them (home, work, auto, etc.) such that you are not at the mercy of the health care system to provide you with this important biologically necessary relief.

Make especially sure that you have baby catheters; size 10 is adequate and not uncomfortable as catheters go. As I mentioned in Chapter 2, the lower the number of the catheter, the smaller its diameter. You should also have Lidocaine or a gel-type topical anesthetic (unless you are allergic to it), a mirror if you're a woman and you need to see "down there," sterile wipes, and a "hat,"[91] or some other vessel to collect any urine that will come out once the catheter is properly inserted into the bladder. Some individuals can self-cath without a mirror and some can self-cath while sitting on the toilet. After all of the time that has elapsed since my diagnosis until the publication of this book, I still have not mastered self-catheterization while sitting on a toilet or without the help of a mirror.

A quick side note regarding the size 10 catheters: If a larger catheter is used on you, the risk is run of creating additional scar tissue in the urethra lining because of agitation with the insertion and removal of the larger catheter. The agitation and/or abrasion can create additional scarring in the urethra lining, thereby making your bladder situation worse instead of better. Go for the size 10 neonatal/baby catheter. "The normal [medical] practice is to use the smallest catheter compatible with good drainage."[92]

It is advisable that you do not leave home without a bladder catheter kit. Since my experience with a total bladder shutdown in November, 2010, I have found it vitally important to carry: rubber gloves, a sterile catheter (which can be washed and re-used), a mirror, a topical anesthetic, a collection vessel, and sanitizing wipes in case a sink, soap, and running water are not available. In this way, I can create my own sterile environment and successfully self-cath without concern for foreign bacteria being introduced into my bladder from environmental contaminants (remember, bacteria can lead to a urinary tract infection).

Keep this kit in the overnight luggage you use. I travel a lot so I never remove my catheter emergency kit from my travel bag. When preparing for a trip, no matter how brief, I just add my clothes as well as shampoo, etc., to my luggage in which my kit is already packed. If there's one thing the Boy Scouts of America got right, it's the motto to "Be Prepared!"

"Sex and sleep alone make me conscious that I am mortal." – Alexander the Great

Chapter 7

Bedroom "Activities"

Fulfilling sex is like so many other aspects of our lives: The "dance" is as important as the end result. For me, gratifying sex begins in my mind. This might hold especially true for people who have Interstitial Cystitis.

Enjoying sexual gratification is an important part of every healthy relationship. Male or female, most of us experience primal intimacy urges that beg for fulfillment. These urges can be difficult to navigate when we are having an IC flare or a full-blown UTI. Nevertheless, there are ways in which we can enjoy our sexuality and have fulfillment despite having IC.

If you are a post-menopausal woman who is still sexually active (as I hope you are), you may need to use a little Premarin to ensure the integrity of your vaginal tissue (estrogens like Premarin must be prescribed by a physician in the United States). Remember that, with age, tissue atrophy occurs and can leave genital tissue fragile and more vulnerable to the friction of intercourse. Friction can be addressed naturally even if your body produces little or no vaginal secretion.

Olive oil holds up well to friction from intercourse and is not susceptible to viscous breakdown.

However, I prefer this water-based 96% organic lubricant (guaranteed pure and natural) called, "Yes WB!" which is available online from the United Kingdom.[93]

Our IC and our need for intimacy necessitates that our partner be sensitive to what we need, what we are coping with, as well as how our health weaves itself into our intimate moments. It is very important that your partner understands what concerns you about intimacy, what hurts you, what helps you, and how you feel sexually at any specific moment in time.

Intimacy must be pleasurable for both of you. As a woman, if you have concerns regarding his cleanliness, then you either need to have a chat with him about his hygiene or you need to clean him yourself. For example, if he is a touchy-feely man and his hands are *not* clean—or his privates, either, for that matter—then suggest he soak his hands (or wash his privates) in a mild, soapy solution and use a little scrub brush to get dirt removed from under his fingernails. I do not recommend a scrub brush for his privates!

There may be *reasons* he has dirt underneath his fingernails. For example, my father was a printer and *always* came home from work with ink under his nails. Your partner could be a mechanic who works with tools and grease, or a landscaper who digs in the dirt...no matter. Again, the point is to be aware and take steps to ensure your health is not compromised during intimacy.

Remember, if his hands or privates are dirty and he is inserting either of them into your vagina, then those germs and all of the bacteria on his hands or privates is being placed *very* near the opening of your urethra, and that can lead to a UTI. Insisting upon his cleanliness is an act of self-preservation—although you cleaning his privates may be erotic for him—so you should feel no shame in having your cleanliness boundaries respected and accommodated.

This should not have to be stated, but if you are not enjoying what you are experiencing when making love, then you must tell your partner what *will* give you the pleasure you desire. Obviously, foreplay, especially for women, is critically important. Intimacy without adequate foreplay will be painful—especially for post-menopausal women—and could very well lead to an IC flare from the friction near the urethral opening. With appropriate foreplay, you should be able to enjoy yourself without apprehension or fear of an IC flare.

Even if you are experiencing a flare, there are still ways to please and pleasure yourself and your partner. Remember when you were young and sexually inexperienced? What did you do then?

Talk to your partner. Be open-minded about exploring different sexual interactions, positions, toys, touches, and/ or self-gratification. If all else fails, be open and receptive to other ideas or redefining what constitutes intimacy between the two of you and, remember, there is much, much more to intimacy than sexual intercourse.

Now, while we're "in the bedroom," let me say a few things about the place of sleep and rest in the treatment of Interstitial Cystitis.

Sleep

Sleep and adequate amounts of resting your body are essential to repairing all manner of internal and malfunctioning tissue damage.[94] Of course, anyone suffering from IC understands that restful sleep can be difficult to obtain because of the many times s/he is up during the night to empty the bladder. People with IC can be up to void as many as a dozen (or more) times a night depending upon that person's individual IC experiences. Interrupting the usual 7- or 8-hour sleep cycle even once can mean that the most restful and restorative part of the sleep cycle—the Rapid Eye Movement cycle (or REM sleep), when dreams occur—will never happen.

REM sleep intervals occur throughout a night of uninterrupted sleep in increasingly longer episodes with the longest episode happening as one begins to wake up—when the bladder is likely to be at its fullest and consequently likely to interrupt the restorative REM sleep cycle benefits.

Repairing and restoring the body is *exactly* what an IC sufferer needs to do, and rest and sleep are extremely important to this "repair/restore" process.

It was recently reported by George L. Bakris, MD, Professor of Medicine at University of Chicago, School of Medicine that "...six hours of uninterrupted sleep per night is recommended..."[95] for preventing hypertension. If six hours of sleep per night can help reduce high blood pressure, imagine what it can do to help you heal your IC. If your IC is like mine was, then you will be extremely grateful to have six hours of uninterrupted sleep (although as your body heals over time, you should be able to increase your rest cycle to accommodate six hours of uninterrupted sleep per night).

Lastly, and perhaps most importantly, understand that the bed (and bedroom) has only *two* functions: sex and sleep! That said, get everything else out of your bedroom which distracts from these two functions.[96]

There is a wealth of information on the internet that can help you transform your bedroom into a haven for restful sleep (see the endnote above and this one for workable ideas).[97]

"All the money in the world can't buy you back good health." – Reba McEntire

Chapter 8

Before and After Interstitial Cystitis

I began to feel *moderately* better after about four months. I shared my feelings of improvement and optimism with my physicians and they were quite guarded, yet hopeful, that the treatment protocol I was receiving from them would heal my bladder. Since these specialists did not know what caused my IC (its etiology), they, like us, are searching for science, data, and testimonials that might provide clues regarding "cause and effect."

My healing was neither a smooth nor a straight road. There were bumps and curves, hills and valleys. I exhibited IC flares that were still quite painful and debilitating but I noticed, over time, my flares were becoming less severe with the approaches shared in this book. Nevertheless, my flares felt like setbacks to my healing, and I often felt like I had taken two steps forward and one step back.

However, about one year after my instillation treatments began, I was feeling tremendously better. My complexion, my skin, my weight, and my sleep were all improving. That is, I was beginning to put on lost weight and catching some REM sleep here and there. More important, my bladder was working on its own and its capacity was increasing—up from less than one ounce immediately following its death to about 14 ounces today. This increase in bladder capacity meant that I could sleep for longer periods of time, again, getting me to that most restorative REM sleep almost all healthy humans experience.

That said, I must share that my bladder still does not work the same as it did before the accident. Here are some "before" and "after" scenarios.

Before IC: An "urge" told me when to empty my bladder.

After IC: I must now be more attentive to what and how much liquid I consume as well as focusing on the sensation of fullness in my bladder to alert me when to "go." The *sensation*, not the "urge," tells me it is time void.

Before IC: I was able to eat and drink pretty much anything I wanted: coffee, soda, orange and pineapple juice, wine, etc., and I didn't have to worry about how it might feel coming out.

After IC: I drink water almost exclusively, and have an occasional glass of red wine, but I haven't eaten or juiced pineapples, oranges, pickles, or strawberries in nine years.

Before IC: I could drink as much as I wanted, of whatever I wanted, and I would only get up once or twice a night to empty my bladder because I had a larger bladder capacity.

After IC: I must not drink too much liquid (of any sort) after dinner unless I can live with the frequent sleep interruptions during the night … and I can't. I value my sleep much more than I value my liquids.

Before IC: I ate almost any type of meat that was put in front of me—including meats preserved with (sodium) nitrates and nitrites—as well as farm-raised fish and genetically modified (GMO) foods.

After IC: I eat only minimally processed and non-GMO foods, and meats that are "natural" or organic containing no nitrates or nitrites, and wild-caught fish such as wild-caught salmon (NOT Atlantic, as the Atlantic is NOT salmon's natural habitat – which ultimately means Atlantic salmon is "farmed"[98] or synthetically produced), swordfish, and cod, etc.

Before IC: I slept through the night uninterrupted.

After IC: My sleep was interrupted multiple times during the night until I rebuilt/restored my bladder's capacity.

Before IC: My bladder capacity was about 17 to 18 ounces per void.

After IC: My bladder capacity *averages* about 12 to 14 ounces per void. After my bladder's complete death, its capacity was less than one ounce per void.

Before IC: I drank a soda or two (usually Dr. Pepper) daily.

After IC: I drink water and herbal teas—NO carbonated beverages. Now that my IC is healed, I have an occasional glass of red wine with dinner, and water-diluted fruit punch from time to time.

"If you think you can do a thing or you think you can't do a thing, you're right." – Henry Ford

Chapter 9

Self-Advocacy

I do not think there is an issue, a diagnosis, or an addiction in America that doesn't have a support or an advocacy group for those who are afflicted. As far back as 1835, Alexis de Tocqueville (no relation), in his classic <u>Democracy in America</u> described the United States as a nation of associations. In your own desperation to find some relief from Interstitial Cystitis you may have participated in such a support group.

I will say at the outset that I am not a fan of "group think" or a "joiner," and so you might want to take the remarks that follow with a grain of salt (not iodized, of course).

My experience with support groups suggests they all have three characteristics in common—all bad. That is, support groups are of no or little help in dealing with the issue to which they are dedicated, whether it be alcoholism, cancer, sexual abuse, divorce, victims of mass shootings, fibromyalgia, drug abuse, mental illness or, of course, IC.

First: All of these groups are based on the conventional wisdom regarding what the problem is, how people normally have reacted to it, and how it should best be dealt with. One of the first things I learned as I approached adulthood so many, many years ago is that the conventional wisdom is almost always wrong. And it's even worse than that: Most recommendations from supposedly well-qualified experts are just as wrong! This is because most people believe what is in their best interest to believe—and they spend most of their lives not listening to arguments *against* what they believe but only arguments *supporting what they have already decided is the truth.* Remember, with IC it may serve you well to keep an open mind.

If you go to an IC group you will be listening to the views of people who have made up their minds about what IC is, how they got it, and what has worked (or not worked) for them. If you have the temerity to suggest they are wrong, you will be shunned, if not publicly ridiculed.

The person who will do the ridiculing reveals the second characteristic of support groups: They are dominated by the strongest personality, the most opinionated person, in the room. Science, whatever there is of it on the subject, has no place there.

The third characteristic of these groups is they become quite quickly a forum for the sharing of miseries: theirs and yours. This results in their members becoming even more discontent about their malady or illness than they were when they arrived for their first meeting. Even the few who achieve some success with their issue—those who choose to share their good fortune—only make the others feel even worse.

While I was collecting notes for this book, I participated in an IC medical focus group that, I am pleased to say, departed from the pattern just described—no doubt because of the oversight and participation by medical professionals who were focused exclusively on the issue necessitating the focus group—IC. I'll take this opportunity to thank them all deeply and genuinely: Each and every one of them were awesome medical experts (at the University of New Mexico Uro-Gyn Clinic), and they include the receptionists who facilitated my paperwork each visit, the nurse assistants who often gave me my instillations as practice for their education-requirement practicums, the nurses who oversaw the nurse assistants, the doctors who diagnosed me and prescribed my treatment protocol, the pharmacists who prepared my instillation concoctions, and even the janitors who cleaned the rooms creating the sterile environment where my treatments occurred. I am grateful to every single one of them.

The IC focus group was composed of women from all walks of life, all suffering from IC. We were asked specific questions about our experiences with IC. As these experiences were shared and discussions unfolded, patients communicated what they wished for—chief of which was that the medical community and treatment providers knew more about the illness. Some participants shared that their IC was so severe it necessitated injections with very long needles directly into the surrounding tissues—which truthfully sounded as if their IC experience was much worse than mine. I was shocked at myself when I openly stated that there were several times during some of my IC flares and the constantly interrupted sleep cycles of a minimized bladder capacity that I actually contemplated suicide as a welcome escape from my suffering: This revelation is directly opposite what I taught my children as their parent, that a minute or a day can make an extreme difference to any of life's situations that may seem completely hopeless. Not surprisingly, other patients also revealed they had thoughts and ideas that ending their life would be easier than continued IC suffering.

In the report that evolved from the focus group, a theme that also percolated to the top was that medical professionals rarely believe patients when patients talk about how debilitating IC is to their everyday life. The cover story of the September 2016 AARP Bulletin, titled, "Warning! How the Health Care System Can Harm You," contained the following remark, "Doctors aren't stupid. They just don't know what they don't know.[99]" Two things doctors will *never* know is how your body experiences your IC pain and how difficult it is, individually, to cope with your IC pain.

When it comes to medicine, most people are reluctant to be assertive with their physicians. The truth is that physicians rely heavily on *you* to provide them with the clues they need so they can provide an accurate diagnosis and an appropriate and meaningful treatment plan. *You* have lived in your body for many years ... your physician has not! Do not be reluctant to speak up and be involved in your own treatment. Physicians also have a duty to share certain information with you that will enable you to take better care of yourself so that you and s/he can work closely as a team.

In the medical arena there are two concepts with which you should become familiar. The first concept is "standard of care." Standard of care means that everyone who has the same medical condition that you have is entitled to the same care or treatment. It is a *standard* by which *everyone* should be treated.

The second concept is a *legal concept that is applied to the medical field and its providers* and this concept is "breach of duty." An over-simplification of breach of duty is the *legal* failure of a physician or health care provider to fulfill the duty of providing you with care that should be available to every/any patient.

It is important for me to state here that I am NOT an attorney and I cannot provide you with legal advice.

The mention of either of those two concepts can send a red flag to a health care provider, health care agency or CEO/ administrators of a health plan that they may have approached a situation which could lead to a medical malpractice law suit. For numerous and very valid reasons, a medical malpractice law suit is something that each of them wants to avoid, just as you should wish to avoid one. Use of these concepts in a written document is never taken lightly. This holds especially true of health care providers, health care agencies, health plans or health plan administrators. These verbal concepts and the use of them are quite serious matters (as you will see in my letters later in this chapter) and should not be leveraged until you have exhausted all other good faith efforts to secure a resolution.

In my case, my "indigent" health insurance coverage ended because my new employer was on a different health coverage plan. This change in health care providers from the one available to me as a less affluent individual to those professionals who were available for me from my newly acquired, job-related health care benefits had tremendous implications for my prognosis: I did not know that I would be leaving the most exemplary female-centric care in the state and descending into the depths of hell with my newly acquired, job-related health plan. But I did!

There are significant differences in female physiological bladder functions from those of males, but with the insurance switch, I went from a highly specialized urology-gynecology clinic that focused exclusively on *all things* female-related to a very basic urology clinic where men and women, adults and children, were *all* treated the same. The urologist at the new health care provider agency informed me on my very first visit that no one at this new facility— not even he as a urologist—had *ever* performed an instillation before the instillation to be performed on me. Trust me, learning this tidbit of information was *not* a confidence-builder! So, I was simultaneously their experimental rat *and* their expert on the treatment procedures and protocol because I had undergone numerous instillations at the previous university clinic, which was now off-limits because of my *new* employment-related insurance coverage.

In the brand-spanking-new urology clinic, I received treatments that were *far* below the standard of care: The physician did not practice sterile technique. This became quite obvious when he washed his hands and put on sterile gloves only to walk across the exam room and open a cabinet while wearing those gloves (which, heaven only knows how many other individuals had opened that cabinet with *unwashed* hands), and then opened my sterile catheter package and inserted my catheter without re-washing or re-gloving after opening the unsterile cabinet door while wearing clean gloves.

Neither did this urologist understand the importance of draining any newly created urine in my bladder *prior* to beginning my instillation (so the medication could bathe my bladder lining), and he used a very large, standard adult catheter, rather than a size 10 neo-natal catheter, thereby agitating my urethra and causing me great pain unnecessarily. During this appointment, I requested catheters of the appropriate size for my next instillation appointment, yet his staff failed to order them as I discovered when I arrived two weeks later for the next instillation.

I was so upset by this inferior treatment that I reached out to a physician-friend who graciously took the time to explain to me the difference between an "appeal" (for a certain outcome such as receiving treatment from a specific provider) and a "grievance" (such as having someone investigated for their technique or for how they treated a patient). Grievances are handled quite differently than appeals are handled and there are also "important legal and administrative distinctions between the two."[100]

Because I wanted to file a grievance for the numerous incompetent actions I was forced to endure by the providers within my new health plan network, in particular from one specific provider, *and* because I also wanted an appeal to receive my treatment from my previous highly competent provider, I wrote an appeal letter *and* a grievance letter.

After several written communications to my health plan went un-acknowledged, I decided to reach out to the plan's CEO. Yes, when I called the individuals who were compensated to answer my questions and they were unresponsive, I decided to take my concerns straight to the top. When you are advocating for yourself, it is necessary that you not be pushed around by anyone. Stand your ground! You have rights to a specific quality of care and, if you aren't receiving that quality of care, the people at the top should be made aware that they have failed in their duties and legal obligations.

Here is my *appeal* letter that I wrote to the health plan's CEO:

> Dear _____:
>
> I regret having to write to you, but after being functionally ignored in my earlier communications with your staff, I feel I must formally appeal to you regarding the denial of continued medically necessary specialty care for treatment by bladder instillation of

chronic interstitial cystitis with out-of-network provider Dr. _____ of [name of clinic].

As you know, under NMAC 13.10.22.8(E)[101] entitled "Out of network services," my [name of] Health Plan is required to allow out-of-network care when the in-network is incapable of providing the specialty care a member requires. While my Health Plan has urologists in its network, I have tried to obtain care from two, both of whom have provided care that is at best questionable and at worst below the medical standard of care. One of these urologists, Dr. _____ [name], prescribed a medically contraindicated medication (name of specific contraindicated medication). The other, much more serious situation that may border on breach of duty is outlined in the attached grievance letter (which has been filed separately as a formal grievance). Because of the unique nature of the procedures I require, and the demonstrable fact that my in-network health plan specialty providers are not trained or conversant in performing this procedure, my health plan network has caused me much distress as it does not have the capacity to provide my medically necessary specialty care.

The data supporting my assertion is contained in the attached grievance letter. I believe that the only way my health plan will be fully compliant with the spirit of NMAC 13.10.22.8(E) as well as relevant NCQA HP Standards[102] is by allowing me to access medically necessary out-of-network care with Dr. _____ [name of doctor] at _____ [name of clinic]. Please consider this my formal appeal in that regard.

Again, I only reach out to you because I feel I've tried every other option and this is a bona fide reason for my health plan to grant my out-of-network request. Thank you for your time.

Sincerely,
[My Signature]

Enclosures: Grievance letter that was sent to my health plan, dated 07/23/14

cc: {To get everyone's attention, I sent copies of my letter to these recipients also:}
Chief Medical Officer (of my insurance plan)
Division of Insurance, Managed Care Bureau (of my insurance plan)
State Representative
State Senator

I am sincerely thankful my health plan took the time to acknowledge my complaints. As my *grievance* letter (ahead) indicates at the outset, I was not anticipating "issues" with my bladder instillation treatments from the medical center at which I was mandated to receive my treatments, so I did not keep a thorough diary of each and every event that took place. (Note to readers: Do NOT repeat my mistake. Do yourself a huge favor and keep a journal or diary of your treatments.) However, I did piece together from the records I kept and I requested that my concerns and complaints be reviewed, then asked that the (below) letter be forwarded in its entirety to whatever peer review panel my health plan used for such matters.

Here is my *grievance* letter (which also served to substantiate my *appeal* letter):

On [date], my first visit to _____ [name of medical center], which came as a referral from my primary care provider, I was to receive a bladder instillation for my Interstitial Cystitis. Upon arrival and check-in, and meeting with the physician, I was informed by the physician that this clinic had never previously performed a bladder instillation. I was asked to sign a medical release form so that my treatment protocol formula (which I had previously received from a provider outside of this health plan network) could be obtained, and that a follow-up appointment would have to be scheduled after the treatment protocol formula was received from my out-of-network provider. *This appointment was unproductive for the purpose the appointment was made (e.g., to receive a bladder instillation) and* *was substandard for that reason, as well as for the reason that the paperwork to obtain the necessary treatment protocol could have been provided to me, completed and returned <u>beforehand</u>, thereby making the protocol available to the provider <u>prior</u> to this appointment and thereby ensuring the bladder instillation would be performed per the appointment pretense.*

On [date], I had to basically educate the physician and his nurse on how to perform a bladder instillation procedure. I explained the swabbing, the catheterization, the draining into a container of any urine that has been produced by the kidneys from the time of check-in and voiding before being placed in the exam room, putting Lidocaine on the catheter, and the breathing technique for inserting and removing the catheter.

I noticed the catheter was rather large and made a mental note to ask them to bring in the appropriately sized (10 neonatal) catheter for my next instillation appointment. Any properly trained urologist should already know that repeated catheterizations with a large catheter can potentially create scar tissue build-up in the urethra, thereby exacerbating the very problem the instillation is intended to treat.

During the procedure on this date:

(1) Swabs were <u>not</u> used independently to clean my urethra opening 3 independent/separate times, from front to back. Swabs were gathered up in a cluster by physician and my urethra was "cleaned" in a circular manner using all three swabs at once. I mentioned the need for front-to-back cleaning with <u>each</u> swab to the physician. Circular-motion cleaning of the female genital opening is substandard care. Using three swabs at once held in a cluster is substandard care. The standard of care for cleaning a female urethra opening is to use each swab independently and wipe front to back.

(2) Lidocaine was placed, in a rather large quantity, on me, not on the first few inches of the catheter (to lubricate it and anesthetize me as it was inserted). *Placing the Lidocaine on the catheter acts as a lubricant. Since catheter was extremely large (in contrast to my very petite physique), not placing Lidocaine or a sterile lubricant on the catheter is a violation of the Hippocratic Oath of "first do no harm" and is therefore, substandard care.*

(3) There was <u>no external container</u> within which to collect any newly produced urine. When I asked where the container was, the physician

replied, "Oh, we will let it drain out on the padding beneath you." Meaning, I was made to lie in my own urine during this procedure! *A department or clinic that, as a routine course of its "medical specialty," handles human bodily wastes should take appropriate measures to ensure patients are not exposed to their own unsanitary bodily waste product(s) during sterile medical procedures such as bladder catheterizations. The fact that I inquired about the container <u>prior to the procedure starting</u> and my inquiry was minimized, <u>and</u> because I was made to lie in my own unsterile urine despite an inquiry that could have eliminated this unsterile condition by not minimizing my inquiry, this matter was handled beneath the standard of care.* At the conclusion of this procedure, I was informed by the physician that these procedures, going forward, would be conducted by the nurse.

On [date], I had an appointment for a bladder instillation scheduled by _____ [name of clinic] for 8 a.m. (I had another business appointment at 9 a.m. at a location about 15 miles away.) I arrived for my appointment at 7:50 a.m. and checked in at 8 a.m. I was finally called back to the treatment room by the nurse at 8:30 a.m. No instillation was received this day and the appointment was rescheduled to a date and time that the clinic could timely perform the procedure. *Making an appointment with a patient and not timely keeping it is beneath the standard of care.*

On [date], and after having a painful/pinch-sensation in my urethra following the first instillation *from the exceptionally large catheter that was used,* and in an effort to ensure that the right-sized catheter was ordered and used going forward, I brought in the catheters that had been used for the nearly two full years of previous instillations from the out-of-network provider. Again, *that* provider instructed me well that one extremely important purpose for using a baby-sized (10 neonatal) catheter is to minimize the chance(s) of scarring the delicate urethra tissue with large catheters on this repetitive procedure.

The nurse performed this procedure. She swabbed appropriately with each swab, independently, cleaning my urethra opening front-to-back three separate times. Other than missing my urethra opening with the first catheter, with the second catheter she was successful and (despite the pain from the large-sized catheter) the remainder of the procedure was unremarkable. *A nurse working in a medical specialty urology environment is expected to know how to locate the urethra and catheterize it. Inability to locate and catheterize the urethra in a urology clinic is beneath the standard of care.*

On [date], upon arrival and check-in, when the nurse called me to the exam room she informed me that the nurse who provides my instillations had telephoned the clinic unwell and that the physician would be performing today's procedure. I asked for my prescription of Bactrim to be refilled. Accommodating my request took a good 15 minutes or more and my procedure was delayed.

The nurse that accompanied the doctor can attest to the following that transpired during the procedure:

(1) The physician gloved, then went to the cabinet above the sink and opened the cabinet, taking something out, and returned to the tray where all of the sterile procedure equipment was stationed. He did not re-glove after opening the cabinet door! *Touching any unsterile object (like a cabinet door that is opened and closed numerous times a day by bare-handed individuals) while gloved and not re-gloving prior to an invasive procedure such as a bladder catheter insertion is blatantly beneath the standard of care.*

(2) The swabs were opened and (just as they were on my first instillation) grabbed in a cluster.

My urethra was cleaned, again, in a circular motion using all three swabs at the same time, <u>not independently and not front-to-back</u> as is the appropriate standard of care <u>for a female patient.</u> *To reiterate from above, circular-motion cleaning of the female genital opening is substandard care. Using three swabs at once held in a cluster is substandard care. The appropriate standard of care for cleaning the female urethra opening is to use each swab independently and wipe front to back.*

(3) An *entire* tube of Lidocaine was squeezed onto my genitals, <u>not</u> placed on the catheter.

(4) The catheter was opened and inserted into my urethra <u>with</u> the instillation syringe attached to the end of the catheter. The catheter is one STEP in the bladder instillation procedure and is not intended to be connected to the syringe containing the treatment protocol, as the bladder must be empty <u>prior</u> to instilling the medication. This 2-step "short-cut" approach the urologist took of not allowing my bladder to drain of any newly produced urine (from the time of my check-in until the time of the actual medication instillation) is beneath the standard of care and is a blatant breach of duty.

(5) The medication was instilled into my very, very FULL bladder (I drink 2 cups of alkalizing tea first thing in the morning, 8 ounces of water, and a 9-ounce glass of juice with which I take my daily supplements). I voided once upon check-in. With IC, my bladder capacity has diminished to about 8 ounces with each void. A full 30 to 40 minutes elapsed from the time I voided at check-in until the time this instillation was received, with recently produced urine thus *diluting* the efficacy of the treatment. *A bladder instillation is medically intended to be given on an <u>empty</u> bladder, not a full one. That newly created urine was not allowed to drain prior to the medication being instilled is beneath the standard of care and is a blatant breach of duty.*

On [date], upon arrival, check-in, and after voiding, this procedure was successfully performed by the nurse. To my complete astonishment, however, I learned that _____ [clinic name] had <u>never ordered</u> the appropriate-sized (10 neonatal) catheter. The nurse did spend a good 30 to 40 minutes attempting to locate a neonatal catheter elsewhere in the clinic, albeit unsuccessfully. Post-procedure up to a week after this instillation, I experienced urethra pain! *Conducting this procedure with a large catheter can cause scarring, and is medically known to cause scarring of the urethra. The [name of] clinic's insistence of using large catheters for the bladder instillation procedure when smaller ones were requested (and a sample of the appropriate-sized catheters was shared with the medical staff, nurse and physician during a previous appointment, and the clinic's medical knowledge that large catheters can not only be unnecessarily and painfully uncomfortable for a petite person but can also create scar tissue in the urethra further exacerbating the problem bladder instillations are intended to treat demonstrated substandard medical care and blatant disregard for the Hippocratic Oath to "first do no harm."*

In sum, I file this formal grievance due to:

(1) Sharing my valuable time, knowledge, and cogent experiences obtained through numerous medically and technically unremarkable treatments from another provider with _____ [clinic name] (and paying my expensive "specialty" co-pay to do so) only to have that information disregarded, as is evidenced by the repetitive demonstrated lack of proficiency with the bladder instillation technique and procedure;

(2) Repeated physician-demonstration of inappropriate cleaning techniques on my urethra;

(3) Physician gloving, touching an unsterile cabinet and not re-gloving before performing an extremely invasive bladder catheterization;

(4) Continued use of extremely large catheters, which demonstrates a glaring lack of patient-centric care; and

(5) Provider inability to *appropriately* drain my bladder of any recently produced urine into an external container *prior* to medication instillation.

Through my bladder instillation treatments at this clinic, I have been the recipient of treatment that is egregiously and blatantly beneath the standard of medically appropriate care any similarly situated patient should expect to receive. Further, I believe this clinic has demonstrated an overt and profound lack of bladder instillation procedure and technique proficiency. My basis for comparing my substandard medical care from this clinic is the 26 previous bladder instillations I received from an out-of-network provider *without* one incident, contrasted to the above-referenced six appointments during which at *each appointment a glitch was experienced.*

I will conclude by asking if the care I received is the type of treatment anyone reviewing my complaints would want for their loved one, their mother/father, sister/brother, or daughter/son? It is precisely this repetitively demonstrated substandard medical care that has eroded my confidence in my health plan's coverage and its network of *specialty* providers. Please be mindful that I pay dearly for this coverage with a payroll deduction from my earnings toward a partially funded employer benefits package, as well as for the quite costly co-pays for *specialty* services.

Thank you for your consideration of these complaints (my formal grievance). I am confident whatever peer review process this health plan uses will agree that some, if not all, of what I have experienced during my brief history of receiving bladder instillations from this clinic are, indeed, beneath the appropriate standard of medical care any similarly situated person or patient would expect to receive from any health care provider.

Under separate cover, I intend to formally appeal for medically necessary out-of-network care as a remedy.

Please feel free to contact me if there are any questions. My contact information can be located on my letterhead.

Sincerely,

[My Signature]

cc: CEO of Health Plan

Medical Director of Health Plan

A few things about the above letters that it will be helpful for you to understand are that there are rules in place which protect you as a patient. Those rules will not do you any good if you do not know what the rules are. Further, each health plan, insurance carrier, and possibly each individual medical provider will have its own set of rules (or standard operating procedures). Learn the rules of the health plan, the insurance carrier and/or the state statutes that cover medical care. Those rules and statutes should be readily discoverable online. It may be a very dry, boring read but these rules and statutes protect you as a patient, and they also protect the various providers as professionals. Learning your options under your state's statutes and under your health insurance provider is your "play book." Understanding the rules, knowing your own body, understanding your IC condition, and understanding the treatments that are available for your IC are the best ways to get a foothold on self-advocating.

Every state has its own rules (and those rules vary from one state to another state) as well as regulations governing insurance and all types of managed care plans. Your state's insurance department and/or Public Regulations Commission will be a great starting place for researching statutes, as well as for discovering a wealth of other important information about your health insurance plan.

I believe I survived by soothing my IC symptoms with resources that are available without a physician's prescription or doctor's office visit. It is these resources—the ones that are provided within this book—that I have shared with you because, as my appeal and grievance letters attest, physicians do *not* have all the answers, despite their believing very much that they do. Which is to say once more what I said at the end of this book's Introduction: In your fight to heal your Interstitial Cystitis, you are on your own!

However, this does not mean you are by yourself. Advocating for yourself will bring you into contact with some members of the health care industry who share your interests and your concerns. It is important, for example, that you understand how "the system" works. As I described earlier, I was forced to deal with "professional" incompetence regarding my IC treatments as a result of coverage changes. (My coverage and standard of care changed when I switched to my employment-related private insurance provider from my previous "free" health care provider.) It was necessary to distance myself from "belief" that these fee-for-service providers—with their Byzantine labyrinth of health maintenance organizations, preferred provider organizations, and private pay mechanisms—knew my health and/or body better than I did.

Consider: Our health care system cannot "decide" the price of a specific procedure. Ask, for example, how much an appendectomy without complications will cost to resolve or, more to the point of this book, "What will a series of bladder instillations cost me?" The potential provider's answer will be, "What insurance, if any, is paying for it?" If you had doubts, know that the United States does not hold the top position globally at providing health care for its citizens;[103] we don't even rank in the top 20 developed countries that provide quality health care. As additional evidence of this you should Google: "United States' infant mortality statistics," or "United States' longevity data," just for starters.

Too many times patients are made to believe that they must accept whatever is dished out to them. Too often patients are intimidated by the health care process. Too frequently we all feel powerless over, and uninformed by, the establishment—the system, the insurance companies, the providers, and their staff—most of which, due to fairly recent HIPAA laws, have prohibited patients' medical issues from being discussed … sometimes even with the patient!

Do not permit yourself to believe that another human being, even one who is well-credentialed, knows your body better than you do.

> "…the most knowledgeable of all physicians who treat women with UTIs, *uro-gynecologists, readily admit they have no knowledge* of the cause, susceptibility, or cure

of chronic cystitis, UTIs, interstitial cystitis, bladder infections...."[104] [emphasis added.]

How can someone who sees you infrequently, sometimes no more than two or three times a year for a few minutes each visit—and then spends much of the allotted time looking not at you but at a computer screen—know your body better than you do? The Internet has made us all equal in ways that some of these elite professionals never dreamed could happen. The products of our medical education system are churning out individuals who are at best semi-literate and at worst glaringly incompetent to carry out simple medical techniques like proper gloving and maintaining a sterile treatment environment – fundamentals that are typically learned in the first year of medical school.

Many Americans have come to realize that being treated by a physician is just as likely to make them more unwell, rather than to help them feel better (or helped) in some meaningful way. This was certainly the case for me with my employment-related insurance provider (sadly, we, as employees, have no "choice" when employers elect health plans for us).

Understanding that you have a voice in your own well-being is paramount. Do not simply hand over your health and well-being to physicians or other health care providers as if those people know you better than you know yourself. The odds are strongly in your favor that they do not know your body any better than you do. *You* have lived in your body; they have not. Our bodies, if we are tuned-in to them, can share quite a bit of information with us. You and *only you*, in turn, can share that information with your health care provider.

For example, if you have an upset stomach, you (not they) will know whether you have eaten something that disagreed with your digestive system. If your IC flares, you (not they) will know whether you have eaten something you shouldn't have, engaged in excessive physical exercise, or participated in an ill-advised sexual practice.

Physicians and other health care providers might have some ideas from their professional experiences about how to help you feel better, but these are only ideas because, as with any disease for which there is no known etiology, the best anyone can offer is conjecture, and the worst is—dare I say it?— complete incompetence. The link between quality medical care and authentic science has proven itself to be extremely questionable if not glaringly non-existent.

"Formerly, when religion was strong and science weak, men mistook magic for medicine; now, when science is strong and religion weak, men mistake medicine for magic." – Thomas Szasz

Epilogue

Hopefully, the information in this book serves to assist you in healing yourself without too much reliance upon the medical community's involvement. There will be, of course, times in your life or health situations that beckon for professional attention. You will be the only one who knows when that situation has arisen and requires that attention. One must be well-tuned to the body and listen to the voice within!

To conclude in a meaningful manner, several readers of this book have already provided cogent feedback that an appropriate ending is "how to select a uro-gynecologist" or other medical professional to assist you through the times when additional medical involvement becomes necessary. This section is intended to provide suggestions which might be helpful as you move forward.

Clearly, there are points to consider as you search for your own medical specialist, whether it is a primary care physician, urologist, gynecologist, or some other professional (e.g., acupuncturist, herbalist, etc.). Here are a few ideas you might consider:

1. Is there a medical urgency to establish a relationship with this practitioner or provider?
2. Is their office conveniently located near you? Will it be convenient to/for you or will you have to endure stressors such as heavy traffic, roads in disrepair, or school- or weather-related delays, etc.?
3. Do they have hospital privileges in the event you need to be admitted into a hospital? If so, *which* hospital(s)? Are these hospitals your medical insurance allows under the plan that covers you and will pay/compensate for services you receive?
4. What is the provider's education? Did they learn from a reputable institution or an institution you've never heard of before? Did they only complete the basic medical education, or are they a specialist?
5. How many years have they been in practice?
6. Are they board certified? Or, do they have other distinguishing credentials that clearly indicate they are well-respected in providing specialty care?
7. Are they proficient in the specialty care and/or procedures you need? This is *extremely* important! (Ask them to describe in a step-by-step process how they will provide you with an instillation, what size catheter they use, etc. If receiving another procedure, ask how that will be performed step-by-step so that you go in with an understanding of what to expect.)
8. Do they accept your insurance provider's plan/ coverage?

9. Will they accept new patients? Many medical specialists worth having already have a full practice and getting in to see them may be impossible.

10. Ask for their Curriculum Vitae or Resume so you may conduct your own due diligence in the form of a background [or fact] check (see 12 below)?

11. Can they provide you with patient reviews? Better yet, look online to see what others say about them without even asking them for their patients' reviews!

12. Conduct an online background investigation or check to ensure they are who they represent themselves to be.

13. Ask them how they will treat your condition, including the treatment protocols and frequency of protocols they intend to use, so there is a clear understanding of what to expect *before* you begin treating with this provider. Stated differently, what are your treatment options?

14. Ask how your condition will be monitored, improved?

15. Are there specific tests they will want to conduct? One of my personal pet peeves about the medical community is that doctors tend to repeat tests that have already been conducted by a previous provider. Ask if they will accept the previous provider's test results to help you avoid additional costs. (Many physicians will want to obtain their own "baseline" of your condition, by way of their own test results and may not accept another provider's test results. You will not know this unless you ask.)

16. What medications do they typically prescribe for your condition (if you know your condition)? What are the

side effects of those medications? Are you willing to endure the worst of those side effects? Remember, oft-times, the side effects we endure are far worse than any benefit derived by taking the medication, some side effects might not even be known or included in the medication package insert.

17. Will you be expected to incorporate lifestyle modifications in order to feel better? (For example, with IC, you must eliminate acidic foods, sugar, and soda from your diet.)

18. What is the contingency plan if the first line of treatment is ineffective (Plan B, and the contingency plan to Plan B, Plan C, etc.)? They should offer you *more than* one treatment strategy! A doctor with only one way or one approach of providing treatment to you may leave you feeling frustrated, angry, and "un-helped."

19. During your first meeting, ask what your disease etiology (cause) is? Then, ask what your prognosis is under their care? What can you expect going forward?

20. Never hesitate to exercise your right to receive a second opinion, or a third!

Appendix A

INTERSTITIAL CYSTITIS DAILY DIARY/JOURNAL*

Date	Beverage Intake	Food Intake	Exercise(s)	Sexual Activity	Results
	How many ounces; what specifically was consumed?	What food(s) did you eat and what quantity of each? Was this breakfast, lunch, dinner, or snack?	Which exercises did you engage in and the duration of time?	Which activities/ positions, etc. did you engage in? Did it create pain or discomfort, or pleasure?	Capture your own self-assessment comments here. How do you feel? Also, capture your urine output here (as measured by your "hat").
Example	12 oz – H20	Yogurt & berries 6 oz	Walking 40 m	Painless Missionary; enjoyable	14 oz pH balanced
Example	6 oz	Steak w/ spices	--	--	8 oz acidic burned

*A daily diary such as this, when taken to your appointments, will help you share your progress and set-backs with your care providers!

Appendix B

Foods that are gentle for IC sufferers:

Almonds

Apple, small

Blueberries

Carob

Cashews

Cheeses, mild (non-aged)

Chocolate, white

Coffee (non-acidic)

Extracts

French sauternes

Garlic

Green tea

Imitation sour cream

Onions

Peanuts

Pears

Pine nuts

Potatoes

Shallots

Spring water

Yellow tomatoes (low in acid)

Zest of orange or limes

Appendix C

Foods that are bad for IC sufferers:

All alcoholic beverages

Apple juice

Avocados

Beer

Bananas

Brewer's yeast

Canned figs

Cantaloupes

Carbonated beverages

Champagne

Cheeses, aged

Chicken livers

Chile/Spicy Foods

Chives

Chocolate, dark

Citrus fruits

Coffee (acidic)

Corned beef

Cranberries

Fava beans

Grapes

Guava

Lemon juice

Lentils

Lima beans

Mayonnaise

NutraSweet (and ALL *synthetic/artificial* sweeteners)

Oranges

Peaches

Pickles

Pineapple

Plums

Raisins

Rye bread

Saccharine (see note above re: synthetic/artificial sweeteners)

Sour Cream

Spinach (*very* high in oxalic acid)

Strawberries

Soy sauce

Synthetic sweeteners

Tomatoes

Vinegar

Vitamins containing aspartate buffer

Endnotes

At the time of publication, all URL links were active. Please note, some entities may remove information or make URL links inoperable. The author has no control over entities referenced herein, or if their information remains available or becomes unavailable.

[1] Silver, George A., M.D. (1987). Public Health Then and Now. AJPH, January 1987, Volume 77, Number 1, pp. 82-88.

[2] Internet Movie Data Base (IMDb). (2000, March 17). **Retrieved May 14, 2019 from** https://www.imdb.com/title/tt0195685/

[3] Alexis, Tracy, PhD (2019). Personal quote. Many physicians and healing practitioners say there is no "cure" for IC. My opinion differs dramatically from theirs.

[4] Nordling, J., Fall M. and Hanno, P. (2012). Global concepts of bladder pain syndrome (interstitial cystitis). **Retrieved May 14, 2019 from** https://ncbi.nlm.nih.gov/pubmed/22057291

[5] Neigh, Gretchen N. and Ali, F. Fariya, (2016, July 29). Co-Morbidity of PTSD and Immune System Dysfunction: Opportunities for Treatment. **Retrieved May 14, 2019 from** https://ncbi.nlm.nih.gov/pmc/articles/PMC4992603/

[6] Colburn, T., Dumanoski, D. and Meyers, John P. (1997). Our Stolen Future: Are We Threatening Our Fertility, Intelligence and Survival? A Scientific Detective Story.

[7] Wang, W., Parker, K. and Taylor, P. for Pew Research Center (2013, May 29). Breadwinner Moms. **Retrieved May 14, 2019 from** https://pewsocialtrends.org/2013/05/29/breadwinner-moms/

8   Cleveland Clinic Health Library. Urethral Stricture Causes & Treatment. **Retrieved May 14, 2019 from** https://my.clevelandclinic.org/health/diseases/15537-urethral-stricture-in-men

9   Look in the "Appendix" section of this book for a suggested daily activities diary template.

10   Harvard Health Publishing/Harvard Medical School (2005, September). Health benefits of taking probiotics. **Retrieved May 14, 2019 from** https://health.harvard.edu/vitamins-and-supplements/health-benefits-of-taking-probiotics

11   Zeratsky, K. for Mayo Clinic (2018, June 18). What are probiotics and prebiotics? **Retrieved May 14, 2019 from** https://mayoclinic.org/healthy-lifestyle/consumer-health/expert-answers/probiotics/faq-20058065

12   Probiotics from Swanson Vitamins, (www.swansonvitamins.com)

13   Probiotics from revital (sic), (www.revital.co.uk)

14   Dr. Gregor Reid Interview, Clarivate Analytics; Archive ScienceWatch (2010, June). Gregor Reid Talks About The Benefit of Probiotics. **Retrieved May 14, 2019 from** http://archive.sciencewatch.com/ana/st/10junProReid/

15   Vitamin C from Puritan's Pride, (www.puritan.com)

16   Cranberry Fruit Concentrate from Puritan's Pride, (www.puritan.com)

17   Finger MD, Mark. (2011, November 11). Renalandurologynews.com. Kidney Stone Prevention: Fact versus Fiction. **Retrieved May 18, 2019 from** https://www.renalandurologynews.com/home/departments/commentary/kidney-stone-prevention-fact-versus-fiction/

18   pH Protector Drops from Swanson Vitamins. **Retrieved June 4, 2019 from** https://www.swansonvitamins.com/q?kw=pH+protector+drops

19   Enzy Medica pH Urine Strips, (https://enzymedica.com/products/ph-strips)

20   The Herb Store, (http://www.herbstorenm.com/)

21   WebMD, Calcium Citrate-Vitamin D. **Retrieved May 14, 2019 from** https://www.webmd.com/drugs/2/drug-32620/calcium-citrate-d-oral/details

22   emedicinehealth.com Calcium Citrate. **Retrieved May 14, 2019 from** https://www.emedicinehealth.com/drug-calcium-citrate/article_em.htm

23   Calcium Citrate & Vitamin D from Swanson Vitamins, (www.swansonvitamins.com)

24 Kilgore, Rachel, DPT, COMT, OCS; Herman & Wallace Pelvic Rehabilitation Institute Blog (2015, October 16). What does Vitamin D have to do with the Pelvic Floor? **Retrieved May 14, 2019 from** https://hermanwallace.com/blog/what-does-vitamin-d-have-to-do-with-the-pelvic-floor

25 Uddin, Rae. The Symptoms of a Vitamin D-3 Overdose. healthfully.com. **Retrieved May 14, 2019 from** https://healthfully.com/295138-the-symptoms-of-a-vitamin-d3-overdose.html

26 Ibid.

27 Anne, Melodie. Livestrong. Is D-Alpha Tocopheryl Acetate a Natural Form of Vitamin E? **Retrieved May 14, 2019 from** https://www.livestrong.com/article/485077-is-d-alpha-tocopheryl-acetate-a-natural-form-of-vitamin-e/

28 WebMD.com. Vitamin E. **Retrieved May 14, 2019 from** https://www.webmd.com/vitamins/ai/ingredientmono-954/vitamin-e

29 Anne, Melodie. Livestrong. Is D-Alpha Tocopheryl Acetate a Natural Form of Vitamin E? **Retrieved May 14, 2019 from** https://www.livestrong.com/article/485077-is-d-alpha-tocopheryl-acetate-a-natural-form-of-vitamin-e/

30 Group, Dr. Edward. (2014, February 14). Global Healing Center. Symptoms of Iodine Overdose. **Retrieved May 14, 2019 from** https://www.globalhealingcenter.com/natural-health/symptoms-of-iodine-overdose/

31 Life-flo Iodine from Swanson Vitamins, (www.swansonvitamins.com)

32 Quercetin Bromelain from Swanson Vitamins, (www.swansonvitamins.com)

33 Quercetin Bromelain overdose. **Retrieved May 14, 2019 from** http://copd.emedtv.com/bromelain/bromelain-overdose.html

34 Patel, Kamal. (2014, January 16). Examine.com. Summary of Quercetin. Primary Information, Benefits, Effects, and Important Facts. **Retrieved May 14, 2019 from** https://examine.com/supplements/quercetin/

35 Dr. Mercola. Food Matters. (2013, July 29). Five Important Ways MSM Could Benefit Your Health. **Retrieved May 14, 2019 from** https://www.foodmatters.com/articles-1/5-important-ways-msm-could-benefit-your-health

36 The Model Health Show. Seven Benefits of MSM-The Miracle Supplement. **Retrieved May 15, 2019 from** https://themodelhealthshow.com/7-benefits-of-msm-the-miracle-supplement/

[37] Answers.com. Can You Overdose on Glucosamine and Chondroitin? **Retrieved May 15, 2019 from** https://answers.com/Q/Can_you_overdose_on_Glucosamine_and_Chrondroitin?#slide=1

[38] Ash, Dr. Josh. Watch: An addition to efficacy of turmeric, helps fight drug-resistant TB. **Retrieved May 15, 2019 from** https://zeenews.india.com/news/health/healthy-eating/watch-an-addition-to-the-efficacy-of-turmeric-helps-fight-drug-resistant-tb_1869683.html

[39] Turmeric. Side-effects. RxList. **Retrieved May 16, 2019 from** https://www.rxlist.com/turmeric/supplements.htm

[40] WebMD.com. Turmeric. **Retrieved May 16, 2019 from** https://www.webmd.com/vitamins/ai/ingredientmono-662/turmeric

[41] Emedicinehealth.com. Calcium Citrate. **Retrieved May 16, 2019 from** https://www.emedicinehealth.com/drug-calcium_citrate/article_em.htm

[42] Everydayhealth.com. Potassium Citrate. What is Potassium Citrate? **Retrieved May 16, 2019 from** https://www.everydayhealth.com/drugs/potassium-citrate

[43] Ibid.

[44] Everydayhealth.com. What is Magnesium Citrate (Citroma)? **Retrieved May 16, 2019 from** https://www.everydayhealth.com/drugs/magnesium-citrate

[45] Examine.com. Zinc. **Retrieved May 16, 2019 from** https://examine.com/supplements/zinc/

[46] Drugs.com. Gotu Kola. What is Gotu Kola? **Retrieved May 16, 2019 from** https://www.drugs.com/mtm/gotu-kola.html

[47] Nordqvist, Christian. Medicalnewstoday.com. (2017, December 14). All you need to know about beta carotene. **Retrieved May 16, 2019 from** https://www.medicalnewstoday.com/articles/252758.php

[48] Sciencedaily.com. Essential nutrient. **Retrieved May 16, 2019 from** https://www.sciencedaily.com/terms/essential_nutrient.htm

[49] Overdoseinfo.com. Overdose Medical Information Destination. Vitamin B Overdose – Symptoms, Dosage, Effects. **Retrieved May 16, 2019 from** https://www.overdoseinfo.com/vitamin-b-overdose-levels-symptoms-treatment/

[50] All Day Energy Greens®, available from Independent Vital Life, LLC, http://www.ivlproducts.com/Superfoods/All-Day-Energy-Greens-Fruit-Flavor-Hi-Octane-Energy-Drink-For-Health-Life.axd?

[51] Webmd.com. Alfalfa. **Retrieved May 16, 2019 from** https://www.webmd.com/vitamins/ai/ingredientmono-19/alfalfa

[52] Elkaim, Yuri. Eleven Life-Changing Reasons to Add Barley Grass into Your Diet. **Retrieved May 16, 2019 from** https://www.urielkaim.com/11-barley-grass-benefits/

[53] Healthline.com. Ten Health Benefits of Spirulina. **Retrieved May 16, 2019 from** https://www.healthline.com/nutrition/10-proven-benefits-of-spirulina

[54] Roberts, Kayleigh. Mindbodygreen.com. Kelp: The Oceanic Plan With Skin, Health & Thyroid Benefits. **Retrieved May 16, 2019 from** https://www.mindbodygreen.com/articles/kelp-the-health-benefits-and-supplements

[55] Webmd.com. Chlorella. **Retrieved May 16, 2019 from** https://www.webmd.com/vitamins/ai/ingredientmono-907/chlorella

[56] Webmd.com. Wheatgrass. **Retrieved May 16, 2019 from** https://www.webmd.com/vitamins/ai/ingredientmono-1073/wheatgrass

[57] Healthline.com. The Benefits of Chlorophyll. **Retrieved May 16, 2019 from** https://www.healthline.com/health/liquid-chlorophyll-benefits-risks

[58] Superfoodplus.com. Blue-Green Algae Health Benefits. **Retrieved May 16, 2019 from** http://superfoodplus.com/ingredients/blue-green-algae-health-benefits/

[59] Webmd.com. Blue-Green Algae. **Retrieved May 16, 2019 from** https://www.webmd.com/vitamins/ai/ingredientmono-923/blue-green-algae

[60] Thegoodinside.com. Nine Powerful Superfoods to Fight Inflammation. **Retrieved May 16, 2019 from** https://thegoodinside.com/9-powerful-superfoods-to-fight-inflammation/

[61] Co-Q-10 from Puritan's Pride, (www.puritan.com)

[62] U.S. National Library of Medicine. Omega-3 fats – Good for your heart. **Retrieved May 16, 2019 from** https://medlineplus.gov/ency/patientinstructions/000767.htm

[63] RxOmega-3, Natural Factors (a Product from Canada), 14224 167th Avenue SE, Monroe WA 98272; also available from Vitamin Cottage and Sprouts (in the United States)

[64] Mayoclinic.org. Omega-3 in fish: How eating fish helps your heart. **Retrieved May 16, 2019 from** https://www.mayoclinic.org/diseases-conditions/heart-disease/in-depth/omega-3/art-20045614

[65] Asprey, Dave. (2015, October 7). Mission.org. The top seven anti-inflammatory herbs and spices. **Retrieved May 17, 2019 from** https://medium.com/the-mission/the-top-7-anit-inflammatory-herbs-and-spices-7c2f88c0644b

66   Agaricus XP Mushroom Tea by Noevir®, contact me at drtracyalexis@gmail.com for assistance placing an Agaricus XP Mushroom Tea order

67   Ware, Megan. (2017, February 23). Medical News Today. What is the nutritional value of mushrooms? **Retrieved May 17, 2017 from** https://www.medicalnewstoday.com/articles/278858.php

68   WebMD. Webmd.com. Cornsilk. **Retrieved May 16, 2019 from** https://www.webmd.com/vitamins/ai/ingredientmono-140/cornsilk

69   Wellnessmama.com. Marshmallow root. **Retrieved May 18, 2019 from** https://wellnessmama.com/15243/marshmallow-root

70   Dr. Mercola. (2019, May 9). Horsetail Tea. **Retrieved May 18, 2019 from** https://articles.mercola.com/herbs-spices/horsetail.aspx

71   ASEA, www.drtracyalexis.myasealive.com

72   Hall, Harriett. (2012, August 7). Science-Based Medicine. ASEA: Another Expensive Way to Buy Water. **Retrieved May 18, 2019 from** https://sciencebasedmedicine.org/asea-another-expensive-way-to-buy-water/

73   ASEA Redox. **Retrieved June 19, 2019 from** www.aseascience.com

74   Wells, Kate. WellnessMama.com. What is the Best Type of Natural Salt? **Retrieved May 18, 2019 from** https://wellnessmama.com/26334/best-type-of-natural-salt/

75   Solaray Magnesium and Potassium Asporotates, https://www.vitaminlife.com/

76   Wikipedia.org. Amino Acid. **Retrieved May 18, 2019 from** https://en.wikipedia.org/wiki/Amino_acid

77   Cohen, Joe. Selfhacked.com. (2018, April 18). Nine Lysine Benefits (Cold Sores) + Foods High in Lysine. **Retrieved May 18, 2019 from** https://selfhacked.com/blog/lysine-health-benefits/

78   L-Lysine from Swanson Vitamins, (www.swansonvitamins.com)

79   Tillery, Enger and Ross. (2001). Essential Amino Acids. **Retrieved May 18, 2019 from** http://hyperphysics.phy-astr.gsu.edu/hbase/Organic/essam.html

80   Webmd.com. L-Arginine. **Retrieved May 18, 2019 from** https://webmd.com/vitamins/ai/intredientmono-875/l-arginine

81   L-Arginine from Swanson Vitamins, (www.swansonvitamins.com)

82   Branched Chain Amino Acids. **Retrieved July 18, 2019 from** https://www.healthline.com/nutrition/benefits-of-bcaa

83   Ibid.

84   Amino Complete, by Now Sports. Available on Amazon. com, Iherb. com or vitacost.com and is also available at Sprouts.

85   Colburn, T., vom Saul, F.S., Soto, A.M. (1993).Environmental Health Perspectives (Abstract). Developmental effects of endocrine-disrupting chemicals in wildlife and humans. **Retrieved May 18, 2019 from** https://ehp.niehs.nih.gov/doi/abs/10.1289/ehp.93101378 and Colburn, T., Clement, C. (1992). National Agricultural Library. Chemically-induced alterations in sexual and functional development: the wildlife/human connection (Abstract). **Retrieved May 18, 2019 from** http://agris.fao.org/agris-search/search.do?recordID=US9545328 and Alavanja, M, Hoppin, J.A., Kamal, F. (2004, April 4). Annual Review of Public Health. Vol. 25: 155-197 (Volume Publication Date 21 April, 2004). Health Effects of Chronic Pesticide Exposure: Cancer and Neurotoxicity. **Retrieved May 18, 2019 from** https://www.annualreviews.org/doi/full/10.1146/annurev.pubhealth.25.101802.123020

86   Chewable Papaya Enzyme, https://www.amazon.com/American-Health-Chewable-Potency-Tablets/dp/B01MRQG8G3/

87   Breath of Fire, https://www.youtube.com/watch?v=SQS4Ad-16vE

88   Womenshealth.gov. Pelvic Floor Prolapse. **Retrieved May 18, 2019 from** https://www.womenshealth.gov/a-z-topics/pelvic-organ-prolapse

89   Kegel exercise, https://www.youtube.com/watch?v=HQDyximQHUg

90   Self-catheterization (women), https://www.coloplast.us/bladder-and-bowel/how-to-guides/female-catheter-guides/; and Self-catheterization (men), https://www.coloplast.us/bladder-and-bowel/how-to-guides/male-catheter-guides/

91   Hat, https://www.vitalitymedical.com/kendall-specimen-collection-hat.html

92   Catheters, https://www.ncbi.nlm.nih.gov/pmc/articles/PMC4673556/

93   Yes WB personal lubricant, https://www.yesyesyes.org/

94   Delucchi, John. Orthocarolina.com. (2018). Sleep: The Secret Ingredient of Injury Recovery. **Retrieved May 18, 2019 from** https://www.orthocarolina.com/media/sleep-the-secret-ingredient-of-injury-recovery

95   Bakris MD, George L. (2018). Insufficient sleep affects BP control in cardiometabolic syndrome. **Retrieved May 18, 2019 from** https://www.healio.com/cardiology/vascular-medicine/news/online/%7B10f12be3-0a75-4974-ba32-9ce9500f8d1b%7D/insufficient-sleep-affects-bp-control-in-cardiometabolic-syndrome

[96] Fields, Lisa. (2008, April 9). For Sleep and Sex Only: 4 Ways to Eliminate Bedroom Distractions. **Retrieved May 18, 2019 from** https://www.health.com/health/condition-article/0,,20189096,00.html

[97] Graven, Andreas. (2012, January 14). ScienceNordic.com. Use your Bedroom for Sleep and Sex Only. **Retrieved May 18, 2019 from** http://sciencenordic.com/use-your-bedroom-for-sleep-and-sex-only

[98] Bittman, Mark. (2009, April 10). The Bottom Line on Salmon. **Retrieved July 8, 2019 from** https://dinersjournal.blogs.nytimes.com/2009/04/10/the-bottom-line-on-salmon/

[99] AARP Bulletin. AARP.Org/Bulletin, (2016, September). Vol.57, No. 7, pp. 18-25.

[100] Appeals and grievances. **Retrieved June 19, 2019 from** https://www.healthpartners.com/hp/insurance/medicare/appeals-grievances/index.html

[101] NMAC 13.10.22.8(E) **Out-of-network services**: In the event medically necessary covered services are not reasonably available through participating health care professionals, the MHCP shall provide in the contract terms that the MHCP and the PCP or other participating health care professional shall refer a covered person to a non-participating health care professional and shall fully reimburse the non-participating health care professional at the usual, customary, and reasonable rate or at an agreed upon rate. The contract must further state that before a MHCP may deny such a referral to a non-participating physician or health care professional, the request must be reviewed by a specialist similar to the type of specialist to whom a referral is requested.

[102] NCQA HP stands for, National Committee for Quality Assurance of Health Plans, the seal of which is a reliable indicator the organization bearing this seal is well-managed and delivers high-quality care and service.

[103] America's Healthcare ranking. **Retrieved June 19, 2019 from** https://www.businessinsider.com/us-ranks-27th-for-healthcare-and-education-2018-9

[104] West, Dr. Bruce. (2018). Health Alert. Miracle Urinary Tract Infection Protocol: UTIs, Cystitis, Bladder/Kidney Infections, Interstitial Cystitis. August, 2018/Volume 35, Issue 8, pp. 1-3.

Printed in the United States
By Bookmasters